MW00325176

About the Author

Ian Wishart is an award-winning journalist and author, with a 30 year career in radio, television and magazines, a #1 talk radio show and more than twenty bestselling books to his credit. Together with his wife Heidi, they also edit and publish the news magazine website www.investigatedaily.com.

Recent Books:

Health
Vitamin D: Is This The Miracle Vitamin?

Global political intrigue
Totalitaria: What If The Enemy Is The State?
Air Con: The Seriously Inconvenient Truth About Global Warming

History
Our Stories
The Great Divide

True Crime
Elementary
Arthur Allan Thomas: The Inside Story
Breaking Silence
Missing Pieces

Dedication

To the doctors, nurses, researchers, scientists, nutritionists and natural health specialists whose tireless work to make a difference, and willingness to question the 'consensus' when the evidence demands it, embodies the true spirit of healthcare and science

Show Me The Money, Honey

Ian Wishart

HOWLING AT THE MOON PUBLISHING LTD

First edition published 2016
Howling At The Moon Publishing Ltd
PO Box 188
Kaukapakapa
Auckland 0843
NEW ZEALAND

Email: editorial@investigatemagazine.com
Web: www.ianwishart.com

Copyright © Ian Wishart
Copyright © Howling At The Moon Publishing Ltd

The moral rights of the author have been asserted.

Show Me The Money, Honey is copyright. Except for the purpose of fair review-ing, no part of this publication may be copied, reproduced or transmitted in any form or by any means, including via technology either already in existence or developed subsequent to publication, without the express written permission of the publisher and author.
All rights reserved.

ISBN 9780994106483

Cover photo by Dreamstime/JohnMorganSmith
Typeset in Adobe Garamond Pro and Soho
Cover concept: Ian and Heidi Wishart
Book design: Bozidar Jokanovic

Contents

Important Notice

What you are about to read is not intended as medical advice for your personal situation, because there is no such thing as a one-size-fits-all solution. If you wish to begin following dietary ideas quoted by doctors and scientists in this book, see your own doctor first to ensure there is no clash with existing medication or an underlying health issue.

If necessary, donate a copy of the book to your local GP and let him or her pull up the medical research listed in here that's relevant to your health condition, and tailor a programme best suited to your or your family's health needs.

Introduction

OR NIGH ON 50 years, we have been told to eat a low-fat, high-carb diet. Fat, we were told, accumulated in our bodies, whereas carbs like sugar were quickly burned as energy. Eating a high-carb diet combined with regular exercise would fuel our bodies with energy easily metabolised during the day. If we were to include fat, it was best in the form of "healthy" polyunsaturated vegetable oils, so we should stop cooking in animal fats like lard, dripping and butter, and use cooking oils and margarines instead.

Accompanying that advice has been a relentless war on salt, accused of "hardening arteries" and all manner of evil.

Yet despite two generations following that advice since the 1960s, we are fatter and unhealthier than we were before. Our lives are prolonged not by good underlying health, but by expensive medical care that ensures fewer people die from chronic disease at young ages. Every day, many of us take a concoction of pharmaceuticals for cholesterol, blood pressure, diabetes, cancer and a range of other modern conditions. We are not so much 'living the dream' as 'surviving the day'.

Those of us not shadow-dancing with the Grim Reaper can often be found popping natural supplements like confectionery, in the desperate hope we can make up for something crucial we might be lacking in our diet, and so delay our date with mortality.

If only it were that simple. Despite all of the above, every single one of us knows someone in perfect health who died of heart failure or cancer. We all know joggers and fitness freaks who've watched their diets like hawks and treated their bodies as temples, but who nonetheless have inexplicably dropped dead.

What you are about to read may shock you, but it represents the current state of thinking in the medical world based on cutting edge research. This book will change your life.

If you are a medical professional reading this, please note that I have deliberately chosen peer-reviewed medical studies from the top journals worldwide (clinical trials where available), and those studies—around 350 in total—are cited in the footnotes of each page. This book is effectively a very large meta-analysis (review of studies) of the biggest controversies in health.

What controversies? That a low fat diet is more likely to kill you than a high fat one. That saturated animal fats are better for you than polyunsaturated vegetable oils. That having low cholesterol is more likely to kill you than high cholesterol. That following the new low salt guidelines being rolled out around the world is more likely to kill you than eating two teaspoons of salt a day. That eating chocolate actually helps you lose fat and get rid of wrinkles. All this and much, much more.

If a little knowledge is a dangerous thing, this may be one of the most dangerous (yet liberating) books you ever read...

1

The Story Of Salt

T HERE ARE MOMENTS in human history that are pivotal to the story of civilisation and life as we know it today. Moments which, to the Albert Einsteins of their respective generations, were sublime triumphs over the immediate problem facing them. Unlike Einstein, who was blessed to live in the time of written records, these predecessors are largely unsung—we know of their achievements because we have built them into our daily lives, but we don't know who they were or why they made the discovery.

The person who invented the wheel in the Middle East some six to eight thousand years ago, for example, did something no other animal has repeated, saving us millennia of effort in transport logistics. It undoubtedly solved the issue the inventor was confronted with at the time, but they could have had no idea the future impact it would have.

Sparky, the caveman who figured out how to create fire, was for a time the most powerful person in the world. Every time you light a candle, think of Sparky.

The discovery of coffee by the Arabs in the 1400s is another that most of us are daily thankful for.

Nobody knows who first discovered the benefits of salt, but what we do know is that by around 5400 BC a town in Bulgaria was already processing salt in large quantities and the city itself was named 'Solnisata', or "salt works".

So precious was salt that the Roman legions were paid a 'salary' which, in its literal Latin translation, meant money to purchase salt. When we eat 'salad' the word refers to the original practice of mixing leafy vegetables in a bowl and salting them.

Back in the cave days, humans received plenty of salt in their diets. Nearly half of one percent of your body weight is pure salt, meaning a 75kg adult will have around 300 grams of salt circulating, equivalent to 60 teaspoons of salt, on any given day.

We lose salt when we sweat, and it is critical to maintain salt levels to keep you alive. In hospital you are given saline solution drips. You can taste the salt when you bleed.

Little wonder that for centuries the average human has consumed around two teaspoons of salt a day (10g). A 5g teaspoon of salt provides around 2000mg (2g) of sodium.

Ancient hunters were meat eaters, and gained their salt from the animals they ate. The rise of agriculture after the end of the last ice age changed our diets. Plants and vegetables don't contain enough salt, and they may also have tasted bland without it.

Settlements sprang up around natural salt flats and rock mineral springs, when locals figured out not just how to harvest the crusty deposits but also how to boost production by boiling water to evaporation point.

Salt was essential not just to diet but to food preservation.

At a time when refrigeration didn't exist, 'curing' meats by salting them allowed families to survive through long harsh winters without having to leave their homes and possessions behind in the search for warmer climes. Being able to stay in one 'home', on one's 'land', changed our nomadic existence and allowed for agriculture and permanent settlements to emerge.

So why, after nearly 10,000 years of deliberate salt production, and during a period where human lifespans have doubled from 40 years to 80 years, have we suddenly declared war on salt?

It's a very recent war. An alleged link between salt intake and blood pressure was first theorised in 1904 in a French study.[1] There was no real proof, but it didn't stop the theory becoming hotly debated during the 20th century.

At issue is not salt itself but its sodium content, which is about half of salt.[2]

"Sodium, like water, is an essential nutrient without which life is not possible, and sodium metabolism is therefore very tightly regulated by an interplay between neurons and peripheral hormones," writes the highly qualified Dr Niels Graudal of Copenhagen University Hospital. Graudal has a double doctorate—he's not just an MD but also has a doctorate in medical science.

He points out in an editorial in the *Canadian Journal of Cardiology* in 2016[3] that it wasn't until 1973 that the first ran-

1 Ambard L, Beaujard E. Causes de l'hypertension arterielle. *Arch Gen Med* 1904;81:520-33.

2 "The terms salt and sodium are often used synonymously. However, on a weight basis, salt comprises 40% sodium and 60% chloride. The conversion of different units for sodium and salt is as follows: 1 g sodium = 2.5 g salt; 1 mmol sodium = 23 mg sodium; 1 g salt = 0.4 g sodium; and 1 g salt = 17 mmol sodium."–Source: "Reducing Population Salt Intake Worldwide: From Evidence to Implementation," Feng J. He, Graham A. MacGregor, *Progress in Cardiovascular Diseases* 52 (2010) 363-382

3 "Population Data on Blood Pressure and Dietary Sodium and Potassium Do Not Support Public Health Strategy to Reduce Salt Intake in Canadians", Niels Graudal, MD,

domised controlled trial of reducing sodium intake from 10g to 5g a day was done, and that showed a beneficial effect on blood pressure. It was 1985, Graudal adds, that the first observational study was done linking salt intake to mortality.

For three decades then, we've been educated through the media and public health campaigns that salt in the diet is evil. If you go to the doctor, one of the standard recommendations is "lower your salt intake".

So much "public health" resource has been invested in the low salt message that the World Health Organisation issued a recommendation that dietary intake of sodium be slashed to less than 2000mg (2g) daily. This, they said, would save millions of lives each year.

New Zealand—one of the most "nanny-state" politically-correct nations on earth and often the first to jump on 'public good' bandwagons—provides an excellent illustration of how researchers appear to accept edicts from quasi-political entities like the WHO as unchallengeable gospel. Observe:

"A diet high in sodium is ranked as the second most important dietary risk factor to health globally according to the Global Burden of Disease Study 2013. The scale of this problem has resulted in "salt reduction" being included in the top five priority actions for non-communicable disease (NCD) control internationally and for reducing NCD inequalities. The World Health Organization (WHO) also recommends a "reduction to <2 g/day sodium (5 g/day salt) in adults (strong recommendation)."[4]

DMSc, *Canadian Journal of Cardiology* 32 (2016) 283-285, http://dx.doi.org/10.1016/j.cjca.2015.08.010
4 "The health gains and cost savings of dietary salt reduction interventions, with equity and

There's arguably an element of circularity involved here. The Global Burden of Disease is a unit created by the World Bank and World Health Organisation, funded not just through them but also the Bill and Melinda Gates Foundation among others. The WHO then issues recommendations based on its findings.

So the New Zealand studies appear to accept as a starting point that the WHO recommendations on the lifesaving need to reduce sodium intake below 2g daily are credible and authoritative. Let's see where that then leads the public health boffins—to health taxes:

"Health-related food taxes and subsidies may promote healthier diets and reduce mortality. Our aim was to estimate the effects of health-related food taxes and subsidies on deaths prevented or postponed (DPP) in New Zealand," says another study.[5]

In other words, having accepted the WHO decree, let's see how it can be enforced on the public. This team of researchers ran computer models on expected public behaviour if a series of "health" taxes are imposed by government. Their computer models (subject to garbage-in/garbage-out data limitations) tell them sodium taxes in New Zealand could save thousands of lives a year:

"A 20% subsidy on fruit and vegetables would result in 560 (95% uncertainty interval, 400 to 700) Deaths Prevented or Postponed each year (1.9% annual all-cause mortality). A 20% tax on major dietary sources of saturated fat would result in

---

age distributional aspects", Nghiem et al. *BMC Public Health* (2016) 16:423, DOI 10.1186/s12889-016-3102-1

5 "Effects of Health-Related Food Taxes and Subsidies on Mortality from Diet-Related Disease in New Zealand: An Econometric-Epidemiologic Modelling Study", Cliona Ni Mhurchu et al, *PLoS ONE* 10(7): e0128477. doi:10.1371/journal.pone.0128477

1,500 (950 to 2,100) DPP (5.0%), and a 20% tax on major dietary sources of sodium would result in 2,000 (1300 to 2,700) DPP (6.8%).

"Combining taxes on saturated fat and sodium with a fruit and vegetable subsidy would result in 2,400 (1,800 to 3,000) DPP (8.1% mortality annually). A tax on major dietary sources of greenhouse gas emissions would generate 1,200 (750 to 1,700) DPP annually (4.0%)."

You can see the nanny state mindset in there—tax everything, even in the name of climate change if you have to.

On the scale of their proposed sodium tax they wrote:

"20% tax on total cost of major food contributors to sodium intakes (bread and breakfast cereals; prepared, preserved and processed meat; sauces and condiments; beef, lamb, and hogget; poultry; and takeaway foods and beverages)."

In a parallel report, another New Zealand/Australia research team helpfully added:[6]

"Also the salt tax would raise revenue (up to NZ$ 452 million/year)."

That's a tax of NZ$100 per year on every man, woman and child in New Zealand, so a family of five would pay $500 a year in salt taxes, or ten dollars a week. And that's just the salt tax.

Extrapolate that out to America, and a salt tax could earn the US government in the region of US$25 billion a year.

In the old game of follow the money, detail like this is important when assessing where "public health" recommendations are leading.

---

6 "Health and Economic Impacts of Eight Different Dietary Salt Reduction Interventions", Nghiem et al (2015) *PLoS ONE* 10(4): e0123915. doi:10.1371/journal.pone.0123915

First, tell them it's unhealthy. Then tell them you are impos-
ing taxes to save their lives. They'll thank you for it.

But what if the WHO and public health campaigners are
wrong? Just how strong is the evidence that salt kills?

Unfortunately, explains Copenhagen University's Niels
Graudal, the hard evidence does not actually support the claims
of the low-salt campaigners. Study after study is showing that
people on low salt diets actually have a much higher risk of
dying prematurely.

Indeed, the community in the world with the lowest salt
intake, the Yanomami Indians of the Amazon, have a "healthy"
low blood pressure as a result of consuming less than half a
teaspoon of salt per day (less than 1000mg or 1g of sodium),
but the flip side to that is their average lifespan is only 40 years.
They are not at war with anyone. They don't suffer from street
crime. There are no road accidents. They have fresh food. And
they are dying young.

The Japanese, on the other hand, have the highest sodium
intakes in the world, averaging 6g a day (three teaspoons of actual
salt). They also have the longest average lifespans (84 years) on
the World Health Organisation life expectancy database.

Regionally, the lowest salt consumers are the African countries. People there consume only 1.5g-2g of sodium daily. The
average life expectancy is between 46 and 63 years—far below
the Japanese and the high salt West.

Now of course life expectancy charts are crude way to link
salt intake when so many other factors are at play, particularly in Africa, but that's where the scientific debate kicks in,
because these issues have been specifically studied and other
factors controlled for.

"The relationship between Na (sodium) intake and mortality is still controversial... randomized clinical trials have failed to demonstrate a reduction in mortality rate," reported a 2014 study that nonetheless surveyed 11 other studies and concluded, overall, that salt kills.[7]

However, the devil turned out to be in the detail.

Five of the eleven studies they surveyed actually found either no evidence of a link between salt and CVD death (two studies), or that in fact a low salt diet was more likely to cause a fatal heart attack (three studies). Buried in the fine print was an admission that 24 hour urine testing was the most accurate way of measuring salt consumption, and that of those studies that did that, none found evidence that salt causes cardiovascular fatalities:

"Contrary to expectations and in accordance with a previous meta-analysis, the studies that assessed Na consumption by 24 h urine collection were unable to find any significant association with CVD mortality."

A 2012 study had shed light on this as well. Researchers suggested that health messages and studies have become too simplistic, with research teams concentrating on narrow points instead of the big picture. The danger of this with salt, they warned, is that the chemical is fundamental to human life and involved in far more bodily functions than just blood pressure.

"Universal reduction in sodium intake has long been recommended, largely because of its proven ability to lower blood pressure for some. However, multiple randomized trials have also demonstrated that similar reductions in sodium increase

---

7 "Daily sodium consumption and CVD mortality in the general population: systematic review and meta-analysis of prospective studies", Poggio et al, *Public Health Nutrition*: 18(4), 695-704 doi:10.1017/S1368980014000949, May 2014

plasma renin activity and aldosterone secretion, insulin resistance, sympathetic nerve activity, serum cholesterol, and triglyceride levels. Thus, the health consequences of reducing sodium cannot be predicted by its impact on any single physiologic characteristic but will reflect the net of conflicting effects."[8]

In plain English? Fiddle with salt levels at your own peril.

They then listed examples of precisely that, including how people placed on low salt diets were more likely to die:

"Three randomized trials have found that heart failure subjects allocated to 1.8 g of sodium have significantly increased morbidity and mortality compared with those at 2.8 g.

"Sodium intakes above and below the range of 2.5-6.0 g/day are associated with increased cardiovascular risk. This robust body of evidence does not support universal reduction of sodium intake."

Remember, the WHO wants us to cut our sodium intakes below 2g/day, and that's a level scientists warn could actually kill us.

The evidence that we may have got it wrong on salt began emerging in the 90s, and grew stronger in the decade that followed.

In 2006, researchers found those taking less than 2.3g/day of sodium were 37% more likely to die from cardiovascular disease, whereas those with higher intakes were not. "The inverse association of sodium to CVD mortality seen here raises questions regarding the likelihood of a survival advantage accompanying a lower sodium diet."[9]

---

8 *Am J Hypertens.* 2012 Jul;25(7):727-34. doi: 10.1038/ajh.2012.52. Epub 2012 May 25. Dietary sodium intake and cardiovascular mortality: controversy resolved? Alderman MH, Cohen HW.

9 "Sodium intake and mortality in the NHANES II follow-up study", Cohen et al *Am J Med.*

A 2008 study comparing those on low sodium diets with those on high sodium found the low-salt people had a 39% increased risk. Every time they checked the data on those with the lowest sodium intakes and those with the highest, they "consistently" found the low salt sample had the highest number of deaths.

Yet try as they did, no data supported a link between higher salt intake and death from heart disease:[10]

"No statistically significant direct association of higher sodium with higher mortality was observed in any comparison."

The study authors concluded that "higher sodium is unlikely to be independently associated with higher CVD or all-cause mortality."

They pointed out that while more than 100 randomised clinical trials—the gold standard in science—have found that salt influences blood pressure, there's no evidence that salt actually kills as a result:

"There are, however, no randomized trial data linking sodium intake to CVD events or mortality."

Yet on the other hand, low salt advocates continue to focus on the links to blood pressure, and invite readers to make the assumption of a link to death:

"Raised blood pressure is a major cause of cardiovascular disease," noted one study,[11] "responsible for 62% of stroke and 49% of coronary heart disease. There is overwhelming evidence that dietary salt is the major cause of raised blood pressure and

2006 Mar;119(3):275.e7-14.

10 Sodium Intake and Mortality Follow-Up in the Third National Health and Nutrition Examination Survey (NHANES III), Cohen et al, *J Gen Intern Med.* 2008 Sep; 23(9): 1297-1302. Published online 2008 May 9. doi: 10.1007/s11606-008-0645-6

11 "Reducing Population Salt Intake Worldwide: From Evidence to Implementation," Feng J. He, Graham A. MacGregor, *Progress in Cardiovascular Diseases* 52 (2010) 363-382

that a reduction in salt intake lowers blood pressure, thereby, reducing blood pressure-related diseases."

In the biggest study of its kind ever done, a massive team of researchers led by Canadian Dr Andrew Mente examined the exact dietary intake of sodium in a sample of 133,000 people from 49 different countries around the world.

Each participant had to provide a urine sample from which their ingestion of potassium and sodium could be accurately measured. The daily intake of sodium was then measured against cardiovascular events and deaths.

Of the sample, 63,000 people had hypertension (high blood pressure), and 70,000 had normal or low blood pressure (normotensive).

The results were published 2016 in *The Lancet*, and have exploded debate across the world.[12]

What they found was stunning. Of the people with high blood pressure, they ran a comparison. Those ingesting the average daily sodium intake in the West of 4-5g (two to 2.5 teaspoons of actual salt) were used as the control group. Then they compared blood pressure patients taking in excess of 7g of sodium a day, and those on a 'low sodium' diet of less than 3g a day.

You would think those on the lowest salt had the lowest risk. Not so. The mid-range 4-5g of sodium a day group (equivalent to 10 to 13g of real salt) had the lowest risk of fatality. Those people with high blood pressure taking more than 7g of sodium had an increased risk of 23%. But those on the lowest amount

12 "Associations of urinary sodium excretion with cardiovascular events in individuals with and without hypertension: a pooled analysis of data from four studies", Mente et al, *The Lancet* online, 20 May 2016, DOI: http://dx.doi.org/10.1016/S0140-6736(16)30467-6

of sodium were at the highest risk of all—a staggering 34% increased risk compared to the 5g group.

It's what the scientists call a 'U' shaped result, where those at the high and low ends of salt intake have a highly increased risk, whereas those taking two teaspoons of salt a day were the healthiest of all.

The results were even more striking for people who *don't* already suffer from high blood pressure. Get this: those of us ingesting more than 7g of sodium a day (three teaspoons of salt) have a 10% *lower* risk of mortality, compared with the control group on 4-5g. But those healthy people with no blood pressure problems who put themselves on 'low salt' diets of less than 3g sodium, were 26% *more likely* to suffer a major health risk within the next four years.

If you are a tofu-eating hipster advocating a low salt diet, you should be really worried right now.

The only people to actually benefit from lowering their salt intake in the entire study were those already suffering high blood pressure and consuming more than three teaspoons of salt (7g of sodium) a day. For everyone else, a low salt diet was more fatal and a moderate to high intake of salt was healthiest:

"Compared with moderate sodium intake, high sodium intake is associated with an increased risk of cardiovascular events and death in hypertensive populations (no association in normotensive population), while the association of low sodium intake with increased risk of cardiovascular events and death is observed in those with or without hypertension. These data suggest that lowering sodium intake is best targeted at populations with hypertension who consume high sodium diets."

Expressed in plain English, the lead authors of the study said in a news release:[13]

"A large worldwide study has found that, contrary to popular thought, low-salt diets may not be beneficial and may actually increase the risk of cardiovascular disease (CVD) and death compared to average salt consumption.

"In fact, the study suggests that the only people who need to worry about reducing sodium in their diet are those with hypertension (high blood pressure) and have high salt consumption.

"They looked specifically at whether the relationship between sodium (salt) intake and death, heart disease and stroke differs in people with high blood pressure compared to those with normal blood pressure.

"The researchers showed that regardless of whether people have high blood pressure, low-sodium intake is associated with more heart attacks, strokes, and deaths compared to average intake.

"While our data highlights the importance of reducing high salt intake in people with hypertension, it does not support reducing salt intake to low levels," concluded lead researcher Dr Andrew Mente.

Low salt diets were dangerous to everyone, he said, but high salt consumption was not: "the harm associated with high sodium consumption appears to be confined to only those with hypertension."

With results like that, it puts the New Zealand salt tax proposal in the spotlight. Far from saving thousands of lives a

---

13 "Low Salt Diets Not Beneficial: Global Study Finds: Salt reduction only important in some people with high blood pressure", McMaster University, Released: 20-May-2016 6:30 PM EDT, http://www.newswise.com/articles/low-salt-diets-not-beneficial-global-study-finds

year, a low salt diet at the WHO recommended 2g of sodium a day level could end up killing thousands in NZ and possibly millions worldwide.

"Low sodium intake reduces blood pressure modestly, compared to average intake, but low sodium intake also has other effects, including adverse elevations of certain hormones which may outweigh any benefits. The key question is not whether blood pressure is lower with very low salt intake, instead it is whether it improves health," Mente said.

Dr. Martin O'Donnell, a co-author on the study and an associate clinical professor at McMaster University and National University of Ireland Galway, said: "This study adds to our understanding of the relationship between salt intake and health, and questions the appropriateness of current guidelines that recommend low sodium intake in the entire population."

New Zealand health researchers, to continue that example, are desperately trying to pitch massive cuts in the amount of salt in processed foods as a way to save money in the health system on the basis of allegedly less heart disease, "net cost-savings of NZ$ 1.5 billion (US$ 1.0 billion)" a year.[14]

Except, if the science they fed into their computer models about the benefits of low salt diets is wrong, then those "savings" could actually become extra costs.

According to Dr Niels Graudal, the computer model (garbage-in/garbage-out) that the WHO based its 2g daily limit on was flawed:[15]

"The model estimated that 1.65 million deaths from car-

---

14 Nghiem et al. *BMC Public Health* (2016) 16:423
15 The Graudal editorial, supra, *Canadian Journal of Cardiology* 32 (2016) 283e285

diovascular causes worldwide in 2010 were attributable to sodium consumption greater than a reference level of 2.0 g/d. However, about 80% of the studies in the dose-response analysis included participants with a high baseline BP [blood pressure], for which the analysis was not adjusted, thus exaggerating the dose-response relationship.

"Furthermore, the authors chose not to include data on hormones and lipids in the model, although these data were published in the same Cochrane review from which the BP data were adopted.

"These considerations could explain why the modelled outcome of the NUTRICODE study (the saving of 1.65 million lives) was not in accordance with the outcomes of studies based on real data, which suggest a mortality increased by about 10%-27% in individuals with a sodium intake < 2-3 g."[16] [17] [18] [19]

Another recent study of 900 heart failure patients over three years shows just how deadly the well-meaning advice to "lower your salt intake" could be. The patients were divided into two groups—those whose doctors had put them on a low sodium diet of less than 2.5g a day, and those eating more than 2.5g a day.

"Patients reporting sodium restriction had a significantly higher risk for...death or heart failure hospitalisation," says

16 O'Donnell M, Mente A, Rangarajan S, et al. Urinary sodium and potassium excretion, mortality, and cardiovascular events. *N Engl J Med* 2014;371:612-23.

17 Mente A, O'Donnell MJ, Rangarajan S, et al. Association of urinary sodium and potassium excretion with blood pressure. *N Engl J Med* 2014;371:601-11.

18 Graudal N, Jürgens G, Baslund B, Alderman MH. Compared with usual sodium intake, low- and excessive-sodium diets are associated with increased mortality: a meta-analysis. *Am J Hypertens* 2014;27:1129-37.

19 Mozaffarian D, Fahimi S, Singh GM, et al. Global sodium consumption and death from cardiovascular causes. *N Engl J Med* 2014;37:624-34.

the study in the *Journal of the American College of Cardiology.*[20]
How much higher? A staggering 83% increase in risk! Forty-two percent of all heart failure patients placed on low salt diets were either dead or hospitalised again within the three years of the study. In contrast, only 26% of patients given a higher salt intake shared such fates.

The research team described their findings as "counterintuitive" to prevailing health wisdom, but said they had triple checked and the findings were real. They too found evidence that low salt intake messes with the hormone system causing dangerous fluctuations as the body tries to cope with low sodium levels.

Far from saving lives, low salt diets turn out to be a highly effective means of population reduction. With heart disease already one of the biggest killers in the world, a low salt diet appears to boost your risk by a further 30% to 40%!

The limitations of the evidence currently used to promote low salt diets are starkly shown (*author's emphasis*) in a *New England Journal of Medicine* commentary on the WHO's work:[21]

"The authors of the ...Global Burden of Diseases Nutrition and Chronic Diseases Expert Group (NutriCode), used *modelling* techniques to *estimate* global sodium consumption and its effect on cardiovascular mortality.

"The investigators quantified global sodium intake on the basis of published surveys from 66 countries and used a hierarchical Bayesian *model* to *estimate* global sodium consumption.

---

20 "Dietary sodium restriction in heart failure: a recommendation worth its salt?" Hummel & Konerman, *JCHF.* 2016;4(1):36-38. doi:10.1016/j.jchf.2015.10.003
21 Low Sodium Intake – Cardiovascular Health Benefit or Risk? Suzanne Oparil, M.D., *N Engl J Med* 2014; 371:677-679 August 14, 2014 DOI: 10.1056/NEJMe1407695

They then *estimated* the effects of sodium on blood pressure in a meta-analysis of 107 published trials and *estimated* the effects of systolic blood pressure on cardiovascular mortality by combining the results of two large international pooling projects that included individual-level data.

"They found a strong linear relationship between sodium intake and cardiovascular events and *estimated* that 1.65 million cardiovascular deaths in 2010 were attributable to excess sodium consumption.

"The NutriCode investigators should be applauded for a herculean effort in synthesizing a large body of data regarding the potential harm of excess salt consumption. *However, given the numerous assumptions necessitated by the lack of high-quality data, caution should be taken* in interpreting the findings of the study."

The number of estimates all strung together in that one WHO study illustrates just how much guesswork contaminates the science on salt. Yet the NutriCode study is the basis of New Zealand research for the introduction of a salt tax, based on the idea that less than 2g/day of sodium is good for you.

The scientific controversy over salt has close similarities to the scientific debate over climate change: an over-reliance on computer models based on theories that conflict with real world data. Computer climate modellers have come in for very heavy criticism in peer reviewed scientific journals in recent years because the climate models have turned out to be wrong.[22]

Naturally, low-salt campaigners are furious at the emerging

---

22 See "Overestimated global warming over the past 20 years", Fyfe et al, *Nature Climate Change* 3, 767-769 (2013) doi:10.1038/nclimate1972 Published online 28 August 2013, and also "Uncertainty analysis in climate change assessments", Katz et al, *Nature Climate Change* 3, 769-771 (2013) doi:10.1038/nclimate1980, Published online 28 August 2013

salt science, and they draw on their fellow computer modellers on climate for support:[23]

"Researchers in the salt space are a polarized, uncompromising and self-serving lot, according to this week's paper by Trinquart et al," writes Australian Bruce Neal. "Those that believe in salt reduction shout it loud from one hilltop and those that don't do the same from another. Neither listens and neither pays sufficient attention to those in the valley below wanting to know whether to salt their fries.

"So how did this happen? And what do we actually know about the effects of salt on health? Climate change is the area of scientific argument best known to most, and there are parallels with the salt debate—not least the two key factors fuelling the argument, an imperfect evidence base open to manipulation and misinterpretation, and strong commercial interests vested in one side of the case."

Neal admits his own "conflict of interest"—he's "Chair of the Australian Division of World Action on Salt and Health," and he also admits his side may not have the "highest grade" evidence to support the low salt argument. But he insists the weaker data still speaks:

"The evidence base for salt is imperfect, but there are nonetheless important conclusions that can be gleaned from the totality of the available data. These conclusions cannot be delivered with certainty, but they have proved compelling for multiple and highly credible organizations. In particular, through the World Health Organization, the United Nations

---

23 "Commentary: The salt wars described but not explained–an invited commentary on 'Why do we think we know what we know? A metaknowledge analysis of the salt controversy', Bruce Neal, *International Journal of Epidemiology*, 2016, 262-264 doi: 10.1093/ije/dyw005

recommend salt reduction to all member states: as do the governments and learned societies of almost every country that take a view on the matter."

And yet, the evidence in favour of a higher salt intake continues to roll in. What Trinquart found in his research was that the low salt camp was acting tribally, ignoring studies that did not fit the preconceived idea that salt is bad.

On the face of it, 54% of the 269 "studies" reviewed by Trinquart's team allegedly supported the WHO's goal of low salt diets for everyone in the world. But when Trinquart broke down those "studies" and concentrated on those based on real data, or 'primary studies', he found the opposite—60% of the actual research either debunked low salt safety or was inconclusive on its worth, yet by far the majority (73%) of policy "guideline" statements and commentary articles endorsed the low salt target, and it was this weighting of the opinion commentaries that was overshadowing the real studies.

How could policymakers be so at odds with the actual evidence? Researcher Martin O'Donnell says policymakers liked to cherry-pick data.

"They found evidence of citation bias, with preferential citation of studies that supported their own particular position."[24]

In other words, the WHO and various government health agencies around the world are influencing the scientific debate on the safety of salt, deliberately ignoring the inconvenient truth that salt is good for you at double the WHO limit. They are flooding the journals with "commentaries" supporting a

---

24 "Commentary: Accepting what we don't know will lead to progress", O'Donnell et al, *International Journal of Epidemiology*, 2016, 260-262, doi: 10.1093/ije/dyw014

low salt target, effectively drowning out the actual research studies showing the opposite. Then they appeal to "consensus".

O'Donnell points out that the world has much more to learn about salt, because we know very little on its "physiological effects on multiple systems (e.g. neuroendocrine, inflammatory and immune) and genetic determinants of salt sensitivity.

"Promoting a message of certainty, despite unclear evidence, creates obstacles to research and may lead to ill-informed policies.

"Second, given the debate in the field, guideline committees should exclude those who have advocated a particular position and, instead, only include independent methodologists and scientists in relevant fields (e.g. nutritional and/or cardiovascular epidemiology). The guidelines committees should also exclude advocates or policy makers, as the science needs to be evaluated without pressures and biases to endorse particular positions."

So what does all this mean to the average reader? O'Donnell puts it this way:

"Reducing sodium intake in those consuming high sodium intake (>5 g/day [equivalent to more than 2.5 teaspoons of salt]), to moderate intake levels (3–5 g/day) is not controversial, as there is general consensus based on the consistency of blood pressure and cardiovascular data. The controversy resides in whether sodium intake should be further restricted to very low levels (< 2.4 g/day), which has yet to be sustainably achieved in any population, which is a range where the effects on blood pressure are modest and there are additional concerns about safety."

The average daily sodium consumption in the West is between 3-5g/day. Only five percent of people sampled in the

2016 study were taking more than that. Most of us then, appear to be in the salt 'sweet spot':[25]

"Although lower intake may reduce BP, this may be offset by marked increases in neurohormones and other adverse effects which may paradoxically be adverse. Large randomised clinical trials with sufficient follow-up are required to provide robust data on the long-term effects of sodium reduction on CVD incidence. Until such trials are completed, current evidence suggests that moderate sodium intake for the general population (3–5 g/day) is likely the optimum range for CVD prevention."

Fine, you may be thinking, 'I can control that'. Actually, you can't. The sprinkling of table salt you add to your meals accounts for only 10-20% of your daily sodium intake. Most of your sodium comes from salt already in food, and with the WHO pressuring governments and multi-national food giants to go low-salt, it's easy to see how a 50% drop in sodium in food could swiftly put you on a low salt diet without you even realising or changing your personal seasoning behaviour.

Don't go racing out to increase your salt intake. If you are not on a low salt diet, then you are probably already getting the western average of three to five grams of sodium a day, which appears to be good for your health regardless of whether you have high or normal blood pressure.

If you are on a low salt diet, talk to your doctor about these studies. Sodium ingestion of less than 3g a day is associated with a much higher death rate—especially for people with hypertension.

---

25 "Dietary Sodium and Cardiovascular Disease", Smyth et al, Prevention of Hypertension: Public Health Challenges (P Muntner, Section Editor) *Current Hypertension Reports* June 2015, 17:47

Remember, most of the salt you need is already in the food—table salt at mealtime is only a small amount of your daily allowance.

As if to underline just how far the science on salt has come, a study on salted versus unsalted nuts found they were equally healthy for the heart:[26]

"Dry roasting and lightly salting nuts do not appear to negate the cardioprotective effects observed with raw nut consumption, and both forms of nuts are resistant to monotony. Public health messages could be extended to include dry roasted and lightly salted nuts as part of a heart healthy diet."

But if you think the revelations on salt are mind-blowing, wait until you discover what they are saying about chocolate.

---

26 "Do dry roasting, lightly salting nuts affect their cardioprotective properties and acceptability?", Tey et al, *European Journal of Nutrition*, online 8 January 2016, http://link. springer.com/article/10.1007/s00394-015-1150-4

2

Life By Chocolate

SOMEWHERE AROUND THE time the ancient Greeks were towing a giant wooden horse onto the plains of Troy, half a world away the Mexicans (or more accurately the Olmecs) were sitting under the shade of a tree, enjoying a siesta, when someone lazily reached up to munch on a bean pod hanging down over them.

The bean inside was simultaneously bitter yet sweet and, shocked at the taste fusion, someone yelled out 'kakawa!' in exclamation.

Today, three thousand years later, we know that bean as 'cacao', or its Anglicised version 'cocoa'—not to be confused with another well known shrub grub grown further south in the Americas that lent its name and leaves to a popular cola drink, and which consigned the native American tribes that discovered it to the ranks of history's first stoners.

By the time of the Mayan civilisation, the story was that chocolate had been brought to earth by the goddess 'Ixcacao'.

Certainly when Spanish explorer Cortes arrived

in the early 1500s, chocolate was plentiful enough to be carried back to Europe as a treasure of discovery, mixed with sugar and vanilla. It was, however, too expensive for all but the high-born. Mass production techniques in the 1800s finally brought the joys of chocolate to the chattering classes, and it has never looked back. For most of that time however, we've looked at it suspiciously: something that tastes so sinful, with rumoured aphrodisiac powers as well, could not possibly be good for you.

Well, those dark days are over.

Chocolate, it turns out, particularly dark chocolate, is packed full of nutrients called 'flavanols':

"Regular consumption of flavonoid-containing foods can reduce the risk of cardiovascular diseases (CVD)," reported one medical science team in 2008.[27] "While flavonoids are ubiquitous in plants, cocoa can be particularly rich in a sub-class of flavonoids known as flavanols. A number of human dietary intervention trials with flavanol-containing cocoa products have demonstrated improvements in endothelial and platelet function, as well as blood pressure. These studies provide direct evidence for the potential cardiovascular benefits of flavanol-containing foods and help to substantiate the epidemiological data.

"In this study, the daily consumption of flavanol-containing dark chocolate was associated with a significant mean reduction of 5.8 mmHg in systolic blood pressure. Together the results of these human dietary intervention trials provide scientific evidence of the vascular effects of cocoa flavanols and suggest

---

27 "Effects of cocoa flavanols on risk factors for cardiovascular disease", Erdman et al, *Asia Pac J Clin Nutr.* 2008;17 Suppl 1:284-7.

that the regular consumption of cocoa products containing flavanols may reduce risk of CVD."

The study was a randomised controlled trial involving specially manufactured 100kcal chocolate bars—one set including flavanols and one with those antioxidants stripped out. After four weeks of consuming two bars a day, the genuine chocolate participants had lowered their blood pressure by eight percent. "Importantly these effects were observed without any adverse effect on weight."

For years government health agencies refused to acknowledge that chocolate could be good for the heart, then in 2014 the European Food Safety Authority caved, issuing this statement:

"Cocoa flavanols help maintain the elasticity of blood vessels, which contributes to normal blood flow".[28]

A study of 20,951 British men and women[29] found the highest consumers of chocolate (on 100gm a day) cut their risk of coronary heart disease (CHD) by 12%, compared with those who didn't eat chocolate at all. They were 23% less likely to suffer a stroke.

A further analysis of nine other studies involving a pool of more than 150,000 people found chocolate scoffers had a 29% lower risk of developing CHD, and cut their risk of dying from heart disease virtually in half, compared with non chocolate eaters.

---

28 "Scientific Opinion on the modification of the authorisation of a health claim related to cocoa flavanols and maintenance of normal endothelium-dependent vasodilation pursuant to Article 13(5) of Regulation (EC) No 1924/20061 following a request in accordance with Article 19 of Regulation (EC) No 1924/2006" (PDF). *EFSA Journal* 2014;12(5):3654. 2014.
29 "Habitual chocolate consumption and risk of cardiovascular disease among healthy men and women", Kwok et al, *BMJ Heart* doi:10.1136/heartjnl-2014-307050

As the *British Medical Journal* noted in a 2016 commentary,[30] "In contrast to the often recommended heart healthy diet, it has perhaps been both a surprise and a delight to many that recent research has suggested that chocolate in both its milky and dark disguises may have a protective effect against coronary artery disease.

"Cocoa has the richest flavanol content of all foods on a per-weight basis including high levels of epicatechin. The health benefits of eating chocolate have increasingly been attributed to their flavan-3-ol content, found in the highest concentration in dark chocolate. Indeed, flavanol-rich cocoa is thought to activate nitric oxide synthesis which could explain findings of beneficial effects of chocolate on endothelial cell function and blood pressure control."

Nitric oxide synthesis is also activated by sunbathing, which could explain why people who sunbathe have lower blood pressure.

In that original 2008 study mentioned earlier, they talked of anecdotal evidence about heart attacks but nothing proven:

"In addition, a very recent publication [in 2008] examining death rates among an indigenous group in Panama known to regularly consume very high levels of cocoa beverages containing flavanols found that deaths related to ischemic heart disease, stroke, and diabetes were all significantly lower than among Panamanians who had adopted a more Westernized way of living. While these studies are observational in nature and cannot substantiate cause-and-effect, they do provide

---

30 "Editorial: Is life longer with a box of chocolates?", Donaldson et al, *Heart* 2016;102:990-991 doi:10.1136/heartjnl-2016-309468

interesting population based data that suggests that the regular consumption of cocoa flavanol containing food products may have important cardiovascular benefits."

Fast forward eight years with a truckload more evidence uncovered, and a 2016 Swedish study of 60,000 men and women backs that up. Those consuming three to four helpings of chocolate a week cut their risk of heart attack (myocardial infarction) by 13% compared to those who didn't like chocolate. "Chocolate consumption is associated with lower risk of MI and ischaemic heart disease," concluded the study.[31]

In 2012, scientists carrying out reviews of randomised controlled trials reported, "In patients with a previous myocardial infarction, eating chocolate twice a week compared with never eating chocolate was also associated with a 66% reduction in 8-y cardiac mortality."[32]

Another Swedish study found a 17% reduction in the risk of stroke, and explained the benefits of chocolate flavanoids for heart health this way (use this paragraph to convince your doctor):[33]

"The flavonoids may reduce the risk of stroke through several biological mechanisms, including antioxidant, antiplatelet, and anti-inflammatory effects as well as by lowering blood pressure, increasing high-density lipoprotein cholesterol, and improving endothelial function. Randomized feeding trials have found that consumption of cocoa beverages, or dark chocolate pro-

---

31 "Chocolate consumption and risk of myocardial infarction: a prospective study and meta-analysis", Larsson et al, *Heart* 2016;102:1017-1022 doi:10.1136/heartjnl-2015-309203
32 "Effects of chocolate, cocoa, and flavan-3-ols on cardiovascular health: a systematic review and meta-analysis of randomized trials", Hooper et al, *Am J Clin Nutr* 2012;95:740-51. doi: 10.3945/ajcn.111.023457.
33 "Chocolate consumption and risk of stroke: A prospective cohort of men and meta-analysis", Larsson et al, *Neurology®* 2012;79:1223-1229

duces a reduction in platelet activation and primary platelet aggregation in healthy volunteers.

"Moreover, randomized trials have shown that intake of high-flavonoid dark chocolate is associated with an improvement in endothelial function, which was indicated by an increase in brachial artery flow-mediated dilation. This dilation effect may be mediated through an increase in local production of nitric oxide. Several short-term feeding trials have further shown that consumption of chocolate or cocoa products decreases systolic and diastolic blood pressure, and may decrease concentrations of LDL cholesterol."

One area of interest to medical scientists is congestive heart failure (CHF), which the common go-to drugs—statins—are "ineffective" against: "alternative therapies are a clinical need," noted one study team.[34] So they chose chocolate. In a double-blind randomised trial, CHF patients taking two bars of chocolate a day dramatically improved their circulation between 20 to 30% based on flow measurement through the brachial artery.

"Flavanol-rich chocolate acutely improves vascular function in patients with CHF. A sustained effect was seen after daily consumption over a 4-week period, even after 12 h abstinence. These beneficial effects were paralleled by an inhibition of platelet function."

Another study of more than 20,000 US male doctors found up to a 40% reduction in heart failure risk for those men consuming more than five servings a week of chocolate, compared

---

34 "Cardiovascular effects of flavanol-rich chocolate in patients with heart failure", Flammer et al, *European Heart Journal* (2012) 33, 2172-2180 doi:10.1093/eurheartj/ehr448

to the lowest consumers, but only if their body mass index was less than 25kg/m2. For those men carrying more lard, it was too much for mere chocolate to overcome.[35]

"The benefits of dark chocolate are better seen in early or intermediate stages of the atherosclerotic process, failing to benefit patients with overt and irreversible atherosclerotic disease. In this sense, we can suggest flavanol-containing cocoa as a promising and powerful option for cardiovascular primary prevention."[36]

OK, chocolate is good for the heart, despite being high in saturated fat[37]. It seems like a contradiction in terms, but it's not a licence to go out and gorge yourself on a box of Forrest Gump's finest—the lesson is one of moderation; at moderate amounts, the useful ingredients in chocolate outweigh the negative ones.

The discovery raised the question, however: does chocolate make you fat? The answer it seems, again paradoxically, is no.

Chocolate appears to increase body metabolism, among other things, which helps you actually burn fat.[38]

"Dark chocolate, a high source of polyphenols, and flavanols in particular, has lately received attention for its possible role

---

35 "Chocolate consumption and risk of heart failure in the Physicians' Health Study", Petrone et al, *European Journal of Heart Failure* (2014) 16, 1372-1376 doi:10.1002/ejhf.180
36 "Central Arterial Hemodynamic Effects of Dark Chocolate Ingestion in Young Healthy People: A Randomized and Controlled Trial," Pereira et al, *Cardiology Research and Practice* Volume 2014, Article ID 945951, 7 pages http://dx.doi.org/10.1155/2014/945951
37 The terms 'saturated' and 'unsaturated' have nothing to do with whether the thing is dripping in fat. Rather, they describe the atomic bonds between adjacent carbon atoms in the fatty acid. Two C atoms joined by a single bond are called 'saturated', those with double bonds are called unsaturated, and those with multiple double bonds are polyunsaturated.
38 Farhat, G., Drummond, S., Fyfe, L. and Al-Dujaili, E. A. S. (2014), Dark Chocolate: An Obesity Paradox or a Culprit for Weight Gain?. *Phytother. Res.*, 28: 791-797. doi: 10.1002/ptr.5062

in modulating obesity because of its potential effect on fat and carbohydrate metabolism, as well as on satiety (the feeling of 'fullness', satiated).

"The research undertaken to date has shown promising results, with the possible implication of cocoa/dark chocolate in the modulation of obesity and body weight."

A study of a thousand men and women in San Diego found people who ate more chocolate were in fact slimmer:[39]

"Adults who consumed chocolate more frequently had a lower BMI than those who consumed chocolate less often. The findings were retained or strengthened in a range of adjustment models and was not explained by calorie intake (frequent chocolate intake was linked to more overall calories), activity, or other assessed potential confounders.

"The connection of higher chocolate consumption frequency to lower BMI is opposite to associations presumed based on calories alone.

"In conclusion, our findings—that more frequent chocolate intake is linked to lower BMI—are intriguing. They accord with other findings suggesting that diet composition, as well as calorie number, may influence BMI."

The key words in there? Diet composition, rather than overall calorie intake, may determine your BMI. Like mother used to say, "eat a balanced diet, everything in moderation", which also fits with the chapter on salt.

To test those findings, a Spanish research team tested 1458 teenagers from ten major European cities. They found high

---

39 "Association Between More Frequent Chocolate Consumption and Lower Body Mass Index", Golomb et al, *Arch Intern Med.* 2012;172(6):519-521. doi:10.1001/archinternmed.2011.2100.

chocolate-eaters were ingesting the most saturated fat, but were also the healthiest:

"Adolescents in the higher tertile [third] of chocolate consumption (median, 42.6 g/d) had lower marker levels of fatness, were more physically active, had higher energy, and saturated fat intake compared with those in the lower tertile (median, 4.7 g/d).[40]

"Higher chocolate consumption was associated with lower levels of total and central fatness, as estimated by BMI, body fat estimated from skinfolds and BIA, and waist circumference, regardless of sex, age, sexual maturation, total energy, saturated fat, fruit and vegetable intake, as well as physical activity. Additionally, when analyses were adjusted for tea and coffee consumption, the results remained unchanged."

Studies like these have an important bearing on the growing problem of childhood obesity—providing schoolchildren with a dark chocolate snack bar for their lunch box daily could satisfy the sugar rush while simultaneously help them reduce weight.

A group of women within the normal BMI range but carrying an excess of body fat were given 100g of dark chocolate (70% cocoa) to eat daily, for seven days. Blood tests confirmed they increased their good HDL cholesterol by 10%, decreased the LDL ratio by nearly 12% and there was an added benefit: "a reduction in abdomen circumference was observed."[41]

Which is better, dark or milk chocolate? The basic cacao compounds are the same for both, but the processing dif-

---

40 Cuenca-Garcia M, et al., "Association between chocolate consumption and fatness in European adolescents," *Nutrition* (2013), http://dx.doi.org/10.1016/j.nut.2013.07.011
41 "Effects of dark chocolate in a population of Normal Weight Obese women: a pilot study", di Renzo et al, *European Review for Medical and Pharmacological Sciences* 2013; 17: 2257-2266

fers and dark chocolate tends to have a higher concentration. Milk chocolate is still beneficial but the addition of dairy fats is thought to lower the absorption of the flavanols in the digestive system, which is why milk chocolate doesn't score as highly in the studies.

"For example, ingestion of 100 g dark chocolate along with 200 ml milk results in a substantial reduction of both total antioxidant capacity and epicatechin content of human plasma, compared to ingestion of 100 g pure dark chocolate,[42] and the reduction is even greater after ingestion of 200 g milk chocolate," concluded one research team.[43]

"It is important for the consumer to know," explains another review, "that dark chocolate consumption promotes more satiety, lowers the desire to eat something sweet, and suppresses energy consumption compared with milk chocolate."[44]

The benefits of dark chocolate kick in from as little as one square a day.

There are several ways chocolate affects us.

"The nitrogenous compounds of cacao include both proteins and the methylxanthines theobromine and caffeine. They are central nervous system stimulants, diuretics, and smooth muscle relaxants," reported Dr Rabia Latif at the University of Dammam.[45]

---

42 Plasma antioxidants from chocolate, Serafini et al, *Nature* 424, 1013 (28 August 2003) doi:10.1038/4241013a

43 "Chocolate and the brain: Neurobiological impact of cocoa flavanols on cognition and behavior," Sokolov et al, *Neuroscience and Biobehavioral Reviews* 37 (2013) 2445-2453 http://dx.doi.org/10.1016/j.neubiorev.2013.06.013

44 "Polyphenol antioxidants in commercial chocolate bars: Is the label accurate?", Vinson & Motisi, *Journal of Functional Foods* 12 (2015) 526-529, http://dx.doi.org/10.1016/j.jff.2014.12.022

45 "Chocolate/cocoa and human health: a review", R Latif, *Netherlands Journal of Medicine,*

"Cocoa mass also contains minerals such as potassium, phosphorus, copper, iron, zinc, and magnesium, which potentiate the health benefits of chocolate. Chocolate also contains valeric acid which acts as a stress reducer despite the presence of the stimulants caffeine and theobromine in the chocolate."

Dark chocolate, in particular, acts like an antidepressant:

"Following 14 days of dark chocolate ingestion, stress parameters in the adults exhibiting high anxiety profiles became comparable with the low-stress subjects.[46]

"Chocolate affects stress levels by prompting serotonin production which is a calming neurotransmitter," said Dr Latif.

So how much chocolate should you aim for? Dr Latif's review suggested 60 grams of dark chocolate a day (approx 9 squares).

In 2013, a randomised double blind controlled trial tested 72 people on varying doses of cocoa flavanols, from zero to 500mg a day, for a month:[47]

"At 30 days, the high-dose treatment significantly improved self-rated calmness and contentedness compared to placebo. This is the first evidence on the effects of cocoa polyphenols on mood in healthy participants. The outcome suggests a possibility for cocoa polyphenols for ameliorating the symptoms associated with clinical anxiety and depression."

The question of why we develop chocolate cravings has also been explored, with intriguing discoveries. Chocolate contains

---

March 2013, vol. 71, no 2, p63-68

46 "Metabolic effects of dark chocolate consumption on energy, gut microbiota, and stress-related metabolism in free-living subjects", Martin et al, *J Proteome Res.* 2009 Dec;8(12):5568-79. doi: 10.1021/pr900607v.

47 "Cocoa polyphenols enhance positive mood states but not cognitive performance: a randomized, placebo-controlled trial", Pase et al, *J Psychopharmacol* May 2013 vol. 27 no. 5 451-458 doi: 10.1177/0269881112473791

"unsaturated N-acylethanolamines" which are a similar to a cannabinoid named Anandamide that is produced in the human brain to create feelings of "heightened sensitivity and euphoria".[48]

A possible explanation, then, for the so-called 'chocolate high'. Then there's dementia:

"Data have been ... promising in elderly participants with increased risk for dementia, where cocoa flavan-3-ol consumption has resulted in improving verbal fluency after only 8-week supplementation (Desideri et al. 2012[49]). In addition, after 2 weeks of flavanol-rich cocoa intake, mean blood flow velocity increased by 10 % at 2 weeks in older healthy volunteers (Sorond et al. 2008[50]).[51]

One final piece of good news to end the chapter on: a randomised double-blind controlled trial using chocolate flavanols in a high dose oral supplement for women aged over 40 found it reversed the visible symptoms of aging, reducing facial skin roughness and wrinkles by nearly 10% within 12 weeks.[52]

"In moderately photo-aged women, regular cocoa flavanol

---

48 "Effects of chocolate on cognitive function and mood: a systematic review", Scholey & Owen, doi:10.1111/nure.12065 *Nutrition Reviews* Vol. 71(10):665-681

49 Desideri G, Kwik-Uribe C, Grassi D et al (2012) Benefits in cognitive function, blood pressure, and insulin resistance through cocoa flavanol consumption in elderly subjects with mild cognitive impairment: the cocoa, cognition, and aging (CoCoA) study. *Hypertension* 60(3):794-801

50 Sorond FA, Lipsitz LA, Hollenberg NK et al (2008) Cerebral blood flow response to flavanol-rich cocoa in healthy elderly humans. *Neuropsychiatr Dis Treat* 4(2):433-440

51 "Phenolic compounds in fruits and beverages consumed as part of the Mediterranean diet: their role in prevention of chronic diseases," Aguilera et al, *Phytochem Rev,* online 20 October 2015, DOI 10.1007/s11101-015-9443-z

52 Yoon, Hyun-Sun, et al. "Cocoa Flavanol Supplementation Influences Skin Conditions of Photo-Aged Women: A 24-Week Double-Blind, Randomized, Controlled Trial." *The Journal of Nutrition* 146.1 (2016): 46-50. doi: 10.3945/jn.115.217711

consumption had positive effects on facial wrinkles and elasticity. Cocoa flavanol supplementation may contribute to the prevention of the progression of photo-aging," the study concluded.

Not only does chocolate make you feel good, it improves circulation and heart health, it may be protective against Alzheimer's, it helps you lose weight and it removes wrinkles. #ChocolateHeaven. The Olmecs were right: it is a gift from God.

You've seen the truth about salt and chocolate, but this next chapter on cholesterol is truly going to change your life.

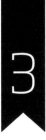

3

Cholesterol, Saturated And Polyunsaturated Fats: Did We Get It Badly Wrong?

W
E'VE ALL HEARD the medical advice on cholesterol. It was first discovered in the early 1800s in the human body, but its molecular structure wasn't known until the 1930s. In the early sixties the American Heart Association urged people to reduce their intake of saturated animal fats in favour of polyunsaturated vegetable oils. By the mid 1980s, scientists were winning Nobel prizes for research into what was swiftly becoming the demon-of-the-day in an era of medical witch-hunts.

According to research since the 60s, higher cholesterol levels mean a higher chance of heart disease, and upon that mantra trillions of dollars in today's money has been invested in health care and pharmaceuticals since then.

In fact, the fear surrounding cholesterol has become so widespread that you can get a thumb prick test done in many malls while you shop, and life insurance companies base their premiums on your levels, among other things.

But what if, like salt and chocolate, medical science was too quick to issue pronouncements on cholesterol last century before it knew all the facts—effectively jumping to conclusions?

That's exactly what medical researchers are now saying: cholesterol has been a pharmaceutical gravy train that never actually arrived at a station:

"The traditional diet-heart hypothesis predicts that replacing saturated fat with vegetable oils rich in linoleic acid will reduce cardiovascular deaths by lowering serum cholesterol," reported a recent study in the *British Medical Journal*. "This paradigm has never been causally demonstrated in a randomized controlled trial and thus has remained uncertain for over 50 years."[53]

It's that last part that is deeply concerning. Fifty years of advice to replace animal and dairy fats with vegetable oils, and still no proof that it works? Even worse than that, there is compelling evidence that people who cut down on animal and dairy have been killed by their choice to roll with vegetable oils. *Not only was the advice wrong, according to new research it was lethal.*

Much of what we know about the animal vs. vegetable issue comes from two big randomised controlled trials done in the 1970s, the Sydney Diet Heart Study and the Minnesota Coronary Experiment (MCE).

---

53 "Re-evaluation of the traditional diet-heart hypothesis: analysis of recovered data from Minnesota Coronary Experiment (1968-73)," Ramsden et al, *BMJ* 2016;353:i1246 http://dx.doi.org/10.1136/bmj.i1246

More than 9,000 people were enrolled in the Minnesota pro-gramme from 1968 to 1973, which covered a nursing home and six state psychiatric hospitals where the participants were long term 'guests'. Because they were eating hospital meals, their diets for the study could be strictly controlled by scientists. Autopsies were performed on those who died—making it the only ran-domised controlled trial where scientists could actually see the results of their diet experiment at a vascular level post-mortem.

The results were as expected. In 1975 data was published at an American Heart Association conference from the MCE trial confirming that 'intervention' diets high in vegetable oils did indeed lower serum cholesterol in the blood.[54]

However, it didn't tell the full story. In 2016 a fresh research team drawn from the US National Institutes of Health, the Mayo Clinic, the University of North Carolina and the University of Illinois (Chicago) re-analysed the mostly unpub-lished raw data collected four decades ago, and ran the numbers with some new questions arising with the benefit of hindsight. What they found literally stunned them:[55]

"Though the MCE intervention lowered serum cholesterol, this did not translate to improved survival. Paradoxically, MCE participants who had greater reductions in serum cholesterol had a higher, rather than lower, risk of death."

How high?

"There was a 22% higher risk of death for each 30 mg/dL (0.78 mmol/L) reduction in serum cholesterol...*there was no*

---

54 "The Minnesota Coronary Survey: Effect of diet on cardiovascular events and deaths," Frantz et al, *American Heart Association Scientific Proceedings.* 1975 October 51 & 52(Supplement II):II-4.
55 Ramsden et al, supra

evidence of benefit in the intervention group for coronary atherosclerosis or myocardial infarcts [heart attacks]."

In other words, the lower your serum cholesterol, the higher and higher you raised your risk of a heart attack.

"Results of a systematic review and meta-analysis of randomized controlled trials do not provide support for the traditional diet heart hypothesis," the study reported.

It's a finding that flies in the face of everything we know about heart health: lower serum cholesterol equals better health, right? Apparently not, and the 2016 study team lays part of the blame on the failure of researchers 40 years ago to publish all the data. If they'd known then what we know now, the advice on animal and dairy fats might have been very different over the years.

There is, they said, "growing evidence that incomplete publication has contributed to overestimation of the benefits of replacing saturated fat with vegetable oils rich in linoleic acid [omega-6]."

The research team found the same failure to analyse and publish all the data in the 1966-1973 Sydney trial as well, with the same result: correctly analysed, diets high in omega-6 oils and low in saturated fat greatly increase (by up to 30%) your chances of dying from heart disease, even though they lower your cholesterol.

"Advice to substitute polyunsaturated fats for saturated fats is a key component of worldwide dietary guidelines for coronary heart disease risk reduction," the study team concluded. "However, clinical benefits of the most abundant polyunsaturated fatty acid, omega 6 linoleic acid, have not been established.[56]

---

56 Ramsden CE, Zamora D, Leelarthaepin B, et al. Use of dietary linoleic acid for secondary

"In this cohort, substituting dietary linoleic acid in place of saturated fats increased the rates of death from all causes, coronary heart disease, and cardiovascular disease. An updated meta-analysis of linoleic acid intervention trials showed no evidence of cardiovascular benefit. These findings could have important implications for worldwide dietary advice to substitute omega 6 linoleic acid, or polyunsaturated fats in general, for saturated fats."

The take-home point, they stressed, is that despite decades of confirmed medical research proving that vegetable oils can lower cholesterol, no controlled randomised trials have ever proven that abandoning animal fats does your heart any good, and now the evidence from such trials says it could kill you.

For decades we've been subjected to the food pyramid. As you've seen, it is being flipped on its head. Suddenly, saturated fatty acids from meat, butter, milk, cheese, eggs, salmon, cocoa butter and chocolate turn out to be better for us as part of a balanced diet than reliance on vegetable oils.

In 2016, a European tong-term study of 35,000 people examined the links between saturated fats and ischemic heart disease (IHD). After 12 years, more than 1800 IHD events had occurred in the study sample—but the long-claimed link between animal fats and heart disease was about to be smashed: higher intake of saturated fats was associated with a 17% *lower risk* of ischemic heart disease.[57]

In contrast, those Europeans who had followed the food

---

prevention of coronary heart disease and death: evaluation of recovered data from the Sydney Diet Heart Study and updated meta-analysis. *BMJ* 2013;346:e8707. doi:10.1136/bmj. e8707

57 "The association between dietary saturated fatty acids and ischemic heart disease depends on the type and source of fatty acid in the European Prospective Investigation into Cancer and Nutrition-Netherlands cohort", Praagman et al, *Am J Clin Nutr* 2016;103:356-65. doi: 10.3945/ajcn.115.122671

pyramid and replaced animal fats in their diets with polyun-saturated or monounsaturated vegetable oils, *increased their risk* of IHD by up to 37%.

"How can this be?" is the question on the lips of cardio specialists whose medical school training and clinical practice has for decades religiously endorsed the "animal fats—bad/vegetable fats—good" paradigm.

A study of 275 patients admitted to hospital after suffering an acute pulmonary embolism is particularly telling.[58] Those with total serum cholesterol approaching 5.0 (average was 4.7), were far more likely to survive than patients whose cholesterol levels at admission were lower (average 3.1).

To put this in perspective, here are the "ideal" cholesterol levels recommended by health officials:[59]

LDL cholesterol: Less than 2.0 mmol/L *
HDL cholesterol: Greater than 1.0 mmol/L
Total cholesterol/HDL ratio: Less than 4.0*
Triglycerides: Less than 1.7 mmol/L

The asterisk in the guidelines goes on to say that if you have heart disease you should be aiming for cholesterol levels even lower than these. So the people who died of their embolisms within 30 days (8.7% of patients) were, by definition, those deemed "healthiest" in terms of cholesterol. The ones who lived were those with "high" cholesterol.

---

58 Association of Serum Cholesterol Levels with Short-term Mortality in Patients with Acute Pulmonary Embolism", Karatas et al, *Heart, Lung and Circulation* (2016) 25, 365-370 http://dx.doi.org/10.1016/j.hlc.2015.09.005
59 NZ Ministry of Health guidelines

In public health discussions, doctors usually refer to LDL as "bad" cholesterol, and HDL as "good".

While you've seen medical specialists argue that lower LDL cholesterol saves lives, the reverse was true in this study. Those who died had LDL average levels of 1.8, while those who survived had LDL at 2.9. The bad turned out to be good.

The HDL figures were 1.2 for survivors vs. 0.9 for the dying, and triglycerides were respectively 1.7 vs. 1.4.

Again, at the risk of labouring the point, the ones who didn't make it were the people with "ideal" low cholesterol.

So strong was the evidence that researchers said they could predict with up to 85% accuracy who was likely not to survive their embolism, based on their cholesterol levels:

"In ROC analysis, total cholesterol level < 3.5 mmol/L predicted mortality with a sensitivity of 83.3% and a specificity of 84.9%."

Similar unexplained linkages between low LDL and a high risk of heart attacks also exist, as the *British Medical Journal* reported 2016:[60]

"That high LDL-C may be protective is in accordance with the finding that LDL-C is lower than normal in patients with acute myocardial infarction. This has been documented repeatedly without a reasonable explanation.[61] [62] [63]

60 Ravnskov U, Diamond DM, Hama R, et al. Lack of an association or an inverse association between low-density-lipoprotein cholesterol and mortality in the elderly: a systematic review. *BMJ Open* 2016;6:e010401. doi:10.1136/bmjopen-2015-010401
61 Reddy VS, Bui QT, Jacobs JR, et al. Relationship between serum low-density lipoprotein cholesterol and In-hospital mortality following acute myocardial infarction (The lipid paradox). *Am J Cardiol* 2015;115:557-62.
62 Sachdeva A, Cannon CP, Deedwania PC, et al. Lipid levels in patients hospitalized with coronary artery disease: an analysis of 136,905 hospitalizations in get with the guidelines. *Am Heart J* 2009;157:111-17.
63 Al-Mallah MH, Hatahet H, Cavalcante JL, et al. Low admission LDL-cholesterol is associated

"In one of the studies, the authors concluded that LDL-C evidently should be lowered even more, but at a follow-up 3 years later mortality was twice as high among those whose LDL-C had been lowered the most compared with those whose cholesterol was unchanged or lowered only a little. If high LDL-C were the cause, the effect should have been the opposite."

Everywhere you look now, the medical consensus on heart health is being overturned as previously "settled" science is found to be wrong.

Take eggs. Well in fact, since *Time* magazine's dramatic 1984 cover story on the dangers of eggs and butter, we haven't been taking them. Eggs, we were told, contain so much cholesterol you were likely to die just from looking at a picture of one.

Yet what have more recent studies shown?

In 1999, a study of more than 120,000 American health professionals and nurses discovered no links between eating high cholesterol eggs, and developing coronary heart disease (CHD):[64]

"We found no evidence of an overall significant association between egg consumption and risk of CHD or stroke in either men or women," reported the researchers. In fact, they found that nurses whose regular diets included an egg every day (7 per week), had an 18% lower risk than nurses who consumed no eggs.

A 2013 analysis of relevant egg studies also found no links between eating eggs and heart disease, unless you were a type 2 diabetic.[65]

with increased 3-year all-cause mortality in patients with non ST segment elevation myocardial infarction. *Cardiol J* 2009;16:227-33

64 Hu et al. (1999). A prospective study of egg consumption and risk of cardiovascular disease in men and women. *JAMA* 281, 1387-1394. doi:10.1001/jama.281.15.1387.

65 "Egg consumption in relation to risk of cardiovascular disease and diabetes: a systematic review and meta-analysis," Shin et al, *Am J Clin Nutr.* 2013 Jul;98(1):146-59. doi: 10.3945/

What's so good about eggs?

"Eggs are not only an inexpensive source of high-quality protein,"[66] writes Julia Reedy of the University of Connecticut for an Honors Thesis, "they contain essential nutrients folate, riboflavin, selenium, choline, vitamin A and vitamin B-12. Carotenoids lutein and zeaxanthin, found in amounts between 200 and 300 ug per yolk, also have positive health implications. Both are associated with reduced risk of age-related macular degeneration (AMD) and may be associated with a reduction in arterial plaque, therefore reducing the risk of CVD (cardiovascular disease). The lipid matrix of eggs also makes these carotenoids significantly more bioavailable compared to when consumed from dark green leafy vegetables.

"Considering the multiple benefits of eggs, coupled with the fact that a reduction of dietary cholesterol results in a reduction of circulating cholesterol in only 30% of people, the apprehensiveness surrounding egg consumption must be re-evaluated. However this cannot be fully achieved in the current anti-fat climate."

Reedy's thesis is fascinating for a whole range of reasons. Firstly, she sheets home blame for the obsession with 'low fat' on poorly designed scientific studies in the mid 20th century. Those studies resulted in the 1977 *US Diet Guidelines*, which became the foundation of nutrition policy throughout the West. Secondly, she points out that although the public moved to 'low fat' food, they ate more of it—partly because it wasn't as satisfying as fattier meals, and partly because the perception of low fat overcame what

---

ajcn.112.051318. Epub 2013 May 15.

66 Reedy, Julia, "How the U.S. Low-Fat Diet Recommendations of 1977 Contributed to the Declining Health of Americans" (2016). Honors Scholar Theses. Paper 490. http://digitalcommons.uconn.edu/srhonors_theses/490

she describes as "consumption guilt" and "dietary schizophrenia":
"Consumers feel virtuous when they eat a low-fat food and
end up overcompensating for spared fat calories; the phenom-
enon has become so common that professionals have given it
a name: 'dietary schizophrenia'."

The low fat foods, packed instead with sugars and carbohydrates as well as artificial flavour enhancers, have seen a
doubling in obesity since 1977 and diabetes. We're eating less
fat, but our health is getting worse. Far from improving heart
health it remains one of our biggest killers despite advances in
medical science and a massive drop in smoking. If unsaturated
fat/low cholesterol diets actually worked, you'd expect to see
hard evidence after 40 years. But no.

The global processed food companies whose products domi-
nate supermarket shelves share common ownership in many
cases with herbicide and pesticide manufacturers, and the big
medical and pharmaceutical companies. In other words, the
investors have found a cradle-to-grave business model where they
clip the ticket when feeding you and also when you become ill
as a result. There are thousands of industrial additives in manufactured food, most of which have never been safety tested.[67]

The overreliance on omega-6 vegetable oils has also reduced
the ratio of vital omega-3 oils in our bodies—the flood of
omega-6 linoleic acid overwhelms the body's ability to convert
omega-3 EHA and DHA lipids.[68]

Naturally, not every specialist agrees with the new research

---

67 *Totalitaria* by Ian Wishart, chapter 6, Howling At The Moon Publishing, 2013
68 "Changes in consumption of omega-3 and omega-6 fatty acids in the United States during
the 20th century," Blasbalg et al, *Am J Clin Nutr.* 2011 May;93(5):950-62. doi: 10.3945/
ajcn.110.006643.

on saturated fats. Adela Hruby and Frank Hu (the lead author of the 1999 egg study) say it depends on what you compare it with:[69]

"The lack of association between saturated fat and CHD in observational studies does not mean saturated fat is benign; it simply means that high saturated fat diets and high refined carbohydrate diets are equally detrimental to heart health."

On the face of it, that's reasonable, except that the Minnesota Coronary Experiment ensured that the only difference between the trial groups was the substitution of vegetable fats instead of saturated fats.

Some studies have found that swapping out saturated fats in favour of unsaturated fats does confer a benefit, but the three studies named in a 2012 review supporting that were done in 1969[70], 1970[71] and 1979[72] respectively, and according to some reports those studies were flawed.[73] Two decades ago, that review of the early work warned:

"The commonly-held belief that the best diet for prevention of coronary heart disease is a low saturated fat, low cholesterol diet is not supported by the available evidence from clinical trials. In primary prevention, such diets do not reduce the risk of myocardial infarction or coronary or all-cause mortality.

"Cost-benefit analyses of the extensive primary prevention

---

69 "Saturated fat and heart disease: The latest evidence," Adela Hruby, Frank B. Hu, *Lipid Technology*, January 2016, Vol. 28, No. 1, DOI 10.1002/lite.201600001
70 Dayton et al. A controlled clinical trial of a diet high in unsaturated fat in preventing complications of atherosclerosis. *Circulation* 1969;40:II-1-II-63
71 Leren P. The Oslo diet-heart study. Eleven-year report. *Circulation* 1970;42:935-42.
72 Turpeinen et al. Dietary prevention of coronary heart disease: the Finnish Mental Hospital Study. *Int J Epidemiol* 1979;8:99-118.
73 "The low fat/low cholesterol diet is ineffective", Corr, L A, and Oliver, M F, *European Heart Journal* (1997) 18, 18-22 https://eurheartj.oxfordjournals.org/content/ehj/18/1/18.full.pdf

programmes, which are at present vigorously supported by Governments, Health Departments and health educationalists, are urgently required.

"Similarly, diets focused exclusively on reduction of saturated fats and cholesterol are relatively ineffective for secondary prevention and should be abandoned."

That was the advice in 1997, and today the issue remains a politico-medical hot potato. All throughout that time the prevailing belief is that high LDL cholesterol levels can kill, but as we saw from the embolism study that's not always true.

Another big 2016 study has blown a hole in the LDL theory big enough to drive a Big Mac through. The research team wanted to know what impact high cholesterol levels were having on a sample of 68,000 people over 60 who, by definition, were more likely to have a close encounter with the Grim Reaper because of their age. If high cholesterol killed, they reasoned, that's where the bodies would be buried.

"If Goldstein and Brown's recent statement that LDL-C is 'the essential causative agent' of CVD is correct, then we should find that LDL-C is a strong risk factor for mortality in elderly people."[74]

Yet when they started digging, headstone after headstone was inscribed, "Here lies a person with low cholesterol":

"The 4-year mortality among those with the highest LDL-C in the included cohorts was up to 36% lower than among those with the lowest LDL-C. Furthermore, in the largest study that included about two-thirds of the total number of participants

---

74 Ravnskov U, Diamond DM, Hama R, et al. Lack of an association or an inverse association between low-density-lipoprotein cholesterol and mortality in the elderly: a systematic review. *BMJ Open* 2016;6:e010401. doi:10.1136/bmjopen-2015-010401

in our study, the risk was lower among those with the highest LDL-C than among those on statin treatment."

That last finding is a shocker: you are more likely to live if your bad cholesterol is high, than if you are on cholesterol-lowering medication.

"High LDL-C is inversely associated with mortality in most people over 60 years," they wrote, meaning the lower the LDL level the higher the mortality rates. "This finding is inconsistent with the cholesterol hypothesis (ie, that cholesterol, particularly LDL-C, is inherently atherogenic). Since elderly people with high LDL-C live as long or longer than those with low LDL-C, our analysis provides reason to question the validity of the cholesterol hypothesis."

It is beginning to look as though serious questions need to be asked about the policy on cholesterol, particularly if so-called "bad" cholesterol actually helps protect against cancer. The war on LDL cholesterol for the past 40 years would explain why cancer rates have gone up.

Cynics have argued that the big pharmaceutical companies get to have a bob each way, making drugs to lower cholesterol that might in turn cause cancer, and then making drugs to treat cancer.

So what do we know about statins and other classes of cholesterol-lowering medication? Do they reduce cholesterol, and do they save lives as a result?

"Early statin trials reported significant mortality benefits," wrote Robert DuBroff in a searing critique,[75] "yet serious concerns have been raised in some studies regarding biased results,

---

75 DuBroff R, de Lorgeril M. Cholesterol confusion and statin controversy. *World J Cardiol* 2015; 7(7): 404-409 DOI: http://dx.doi.org/10.4330/wjc.v7.i7.404

premature trial terminations, under reporting of adverse events, high numbers of patients lost to follow-up and oversight by the pharmaceutical company sponsor.

"Heightened awareness within the scientific community regarding problems in clinical trial conduct and analysis—exemplified by the unreported risk of heart attacks in patients taking the pain killers Vioxx and Celebrex—led to new regulatory rules for clinical trials in 2005.

"Curiously," says DuBroff, "statin trials conducted after 2005 have failed to demonstrate a consistent mortality benefit."

So the first part of the rhetorical question has undoubtedly been answered: these drugs do reduce LDL cholesterol levels. But if you've been following this chapter closely on the dangers of low cholesterol, you will be hearing alarm bells going off. Right about now:

"Eli Lilly said on Monday that it was halting development of a drug for cardiovascular disease because the drug was not likely to be found effective in preventing heart attacks and strokes," wrote *New York Times* journalist Andrew Pollack in late 2015.[76]

"The move is a blow for Lilly; the drug, evacetrapib, was in the final stage of clinical trials and was expected to become a blockbuster had it reached the market.

"It is also the latest disappointment for this class of drugs, known as CETP inhibitors, which can raise the levels of so-called good cholesterol while lowering the levels of bad cholesterol.

"Pfizer halted a late-stage study of its CETP inhibitor, torce-

---

76 Eli Lilly Abandons Heart Disease Drug in Final Stage of Trials By ANDREW POLLACK ,NYT, OCT. 12, 2015

trapib, in late 2006, when the drug, despite raising good cholesterol levels as intended, was found to increase the risk of death and heart problems in a clinical trial. Roche gave up on its candidate, dalcetrapib, in 2012, after a trial suggested the drug was not effective."

The next chapter in that horror story came in April 2016 when Eli Lilly revealed the full findings of its clinical trial. Again, the *New York Times*:[77]

"It is a drug that reduces levels of LDL cholesterol, the dangerous kind, as much as statins do. And it more than doubles levels of HDL cholesterol, the good kind, which is linked to protection from heart disease. As a result, heart experts had high hopes for it as an alternative for the many patients who cannot or will not take statins.

"But these specialists were stunned by the results of a study of 12,000 patients, announced on Sunday at the American College of Cardiology's annual meeting: There was no benefit from taking the drug, evacetrapib. The drug's maker, Eli Lilly, stopped the study in October, citing futility, but it was not until Sunday's meeting that cardiologists first saw the data behind that decision.

"Participants taking the drug saw their LDL levels fall to an average of 55 milligrams per deciliter from 84. Their HDL levels rose to an average of 104 milligram per deciliter from 46. Yet 256 participants had heart attacks, compared with 255 patients in the group who were taking a placebo. Ninety-two patients taking the drug had a stroke, compared with 95 in

---

77 "Dashing hopes, study shows cholesterol drug had no effect on heart health" By Gina Kolata, NYT, APR. 3, 2016

the placebo group. And 434 people taking the drug died from cardiovascular disease, such as a heart attack or a stroke, compared with 444 participants who were taking a placebo.

" 'We had an agent that seemed to do all the right things,' said Dr. Stephen J. Nicholls, the study's principal investigator and the deputy director of the South Australian Health and Medical Research Institute in Adelaide. 'It's the most mind-boggling question. How can a drug that lowers something that is associated with benefit not show any benefit?' he said, referring to the 37 percent drop in LDL levels with the drug."

That, of course, is the $64 million question, even though the answer may be staring them in the face: if cholesterol theory is wrong, then the treatments may be simply expensive urine, or worse. The drug lowered the so called "bad" cholesterol, but it had no impact on CVD. That strongly suggests cholesterol theory is indeed somehow wrong.

Which is exactly the furious debate that's broken out in medical research circles.

A big Japanese study following 7,000 people for 20 years revealed that increasing the level of 'good' cholesterol, HDL, was found to reduce your chances of developing heart disease but had no impact on mortality: "No significant association was observed between HDL-C and all-cause mortality."[78]

So lowering the bad cholesterol doesn't save you, and raising the good cholesterol doesn't either. Both those findings fly in the face of traditional medical advice.

---

78 "The Relationship between Very High Levels of Serum High-Density Lipoprotein Cholesterol and Cause-Specific Mortality in a 20-Year Follow-Up Study of Japanese General Population," Hirata et al, *Journal of Atherosclerosis and Thrombosis* Article ID: 33449 http://doi.org/10.5551/jat.33449

In 2014 yet another research study of 650,000 people found no link between eating saturated fats and coronary heart disease:[79]

"Current evidence does not clearly support cardiovascular guidelines that encourage high consumption of polyunsaturated fatty acids and low consumption of total saturated fats."

The review looked at 49 different observational studies and 27 randomised controlled trials and found the coronary risk from intake of different dietary fats (omega-3, omega-6, saturated fats) was essentially the same—saturated fats were no better or worse for you than vegetable oils.

Sensing a threat to the foundations of New Zealand's healthy policy guidelines, a research team from the University of Otago swiftly went on the attack:[80]

"The finding of no link between fat intakes and coronary outcomes by Chowdhury et al. is likely to be confounded by other nutrient intakes, particularly carbohydrate, for which there has been no adjustment.

"A rather different result emerges when considering also the nutrients which replace saturated fat (as would be the case in real life) rather than individual nutrients in isolation. The review by Jakobsen et al (2009)[81] did just that in a meta-analysis of studies in which individual participant data was

---

79 "Association of dietary, circulating, and supplement fatty acids with coronary risk: a systematic review and meta-analysis," Chowdhury et al, *Ann Intern Med.* 2014 Mar 18;160(6):398-406. doi: 10.7326/M13-1788.
80 Te Morenga L, McLean R, Skeaff M, Mann J. Advice to reduce total and saturated fat, revisited [editorial]. *N Z Med J.* 2014;127(1392):12-16. http://journal.nzma.org.nz/journal/127-1392/6078/content.pdf
81 Jakobsen MU, O'Reilly EJ, Heitmann BL, et al. Major types of dietary fat and risk of coronary heart disease: a pooled analysis of 11 cohort studies. *The American Journal of Clinical Nutrition.* 2009;89(5):1425-32.

used as distinct from other meta-analyses based on aggregated study results.

"They found that substitution of 5% of energy from SFA with 5% of energy from PUFA was associated with a 26% reduction in risk of coronary death based on 2155 deaths amongst 344,696 subjects followed-up for 4–10 years. Substitution of SFA with carbohydrate or MUFA was not associated with benefit.

"A meta-analysis of prospective cohort studies involving over 900,000 adults shows a linear association between blood cholesterol concentrations and CHD mortality."[82]

But if that's accurate, how do we explain this comment from another group of scientists?

"Numerous trials of cholesterol lowering have failed to demonstrate consistent benefit."[83]

It turns out that—in the same way as we saw in the salt chapter—supporters of the "establishment" view are being accused of cherrypicking which studies they take notice of.

"[There is] some evidence of publication bias. That is that small studies which showed harm from saturated fat replacement were unlikely to be published."[84]

That's not good enough, say critics, because if cholesterol theory is true, it actually has to withstand scrutiny and come up with better answers than "unexplained" and the benefits of lower cholesterol should be obvious:

---

82 Prospective Studies Collaboration. Blood cholesterol and vascular mortality by age, sex, and blood pressure: a meta-analysis of individual data from 61 prospective studies with 55 000 vascular deaths. *Lancet* 2007; 370: 1829-39.

83 "Does IMPROVE-IT prove it?", Robert DuBroff, *Preventive Medicine* Volume 85, April 2016, Pages 32-35 doi:10.1016/j.ypmed.2016.01.004

84 "Chewing the saturated fat: should we or shouldn't we?", Thornley et al, *NZMJ* 23 May 2014, Vol 127 No 1394, pp 94-96

"Many physicians tend to ignore the numerous clinical studies which have failed to demonstrate a benefit of cholesterol lowering. This article challenges the cholesterol hypothesis by reviewing these negative studies and our reluctance to acknowledge them. Paradoxically, cholesterol lowering remains the focus of cardiovascular disease prevention despite the inconsistent benefit demonstrated in dozens of clinical trials. The cholesterol-lowering, statin-centric approach to cardiovascular disease prevention may in fact distract us from other beneficial therapies."

The debate, as you can see, is polarising. Go back a couple of paragraphs to the Otago University endorsement of a 900,000 strong study allegedly showing clear links between cholesterol and mortality.

Not so fast. Here's what that big study also found:[85]

"Total cholesterol was weakly positively related to ischaemic and total stroke mortality in early middle age (40-59 years), but this finding could be largely or wholly accounted for by the association of cholesterol with blood pressure."

That's hardly a ringing endorsement. But it gets worse. Take a look at the fine print:

"Moreover, a positive relation was seen *only* in middle age and *only* in those with below-average blood pressure; at older ages (70-89 years) and, particularly, for those with systolic blood pressure over about 145 mm Hg, total cholesterol was *negatively* related to haemorrhagic and total stroke mortality."

As another study in 2016 reported, most of the people hav-

---

85 Prospective Studies Collaboration. Blood cholesterol and vascular mortality by age, sex, and blood pressure: a meta-analysis of individual data from 61 prospective studies with 55 000 vascular deaths. *Lancet* 2007; 370: 1829-39.

ing heart attacks are the 'healthy' ones with low cholesterol:[86]
"Even more striking is the observation that two thirds of
people admitted for acute coronary events suffer from the
metabolic syndrome, but 75% of these exhibit completely
normal TC and low-density lipoprotein-cholesterol (LDLC)
concentrations[87]."

While the public go about their daily lives following traditional medical advice in blissful ignorance, many doctors are
abandoning the idea that cholesterol levels or saturated fat
intakes are relevant any more.

"The global prevalence of CHD, despite worldwide statin
usage and cholesterol lowering campaigns, has reached pan-
demic proportions", warned Robert DuBroff. "Coronary heart
disease is an extremely complex malady and the expectation
that it could be prevented or eliminated by simply reducing
cholesterol appears unfounded."[88]

In the *Lancet*, a group of American medical researchers
warned that lower cholesterol might reduce heart deaths but
increase cancer and other fatal diseases:[89]

"It might result from an increase in both cancer and non-
cardiovascular mortality with lower cholesterol concentrations.
A meta-analysis of large prospective randomised statin trials
showed an inverse relation between achieved LDL choles-

---

86 B. Ruiz-Núñez et al. / *Journal of Nutritional Biochemistry* 36 (2016) 1-20
87 Sachdeva A, Cannon C, Deedwania P, Labresh K, Smith S, Dai D, et al. Lipid levels in patients hospitalized with coronary artery disease: an analysis of 136,905 hospitalizations in get with the guidelines. *Am Heart J* 2009;157:111-7 [e2].
88 DuBroff R, de Lorgeril M. Cholesterol confusion and statin controversy. *World J Cardiol* 2015; 7(7): 404-409 DOI: http://dx.doi.org/10.4330/wjc.v7.i7.404
89 "Cholesterol, statins, and mortality," Goldstein et al, *The Lancet* Vol 371 April 5, 2008, p1161

terol concentrations and cancer risk in statin-treated patients (p=0·009)."

Doctors suspect statins impact on the body's immune system, either by suppressing it or alternatively by lowering the cholesterol normally used by the immune system, "leading to increased cancer risk, particularly in elderly people, since they are more apt to harbour cancer cells. Indeed, in the PROSPER trial, the statin-treated patients had a significant increase in cancer incidence, leaving all-cause mortality unchanged.

"Therefore, there are data suggesting that lower cholesterol concentrations are not always better."

If you doubt a cancer link, consider this from the *Journal of Clinical Oncology*:[90]

"At least nine studies have shown that cancer is associated with low cholesterol, measured 10 to > 30 years before diagnosis.

"Several cholesterol-lowering drugs, including statins, have been found to be carcinogenic in rodents in doses that produce blood concentrations of the drugs similar to those attained in treating patients.[91] In accordance, breast cancer occurred in 12 of 286 women in the treatment group of the CARE (Cholesterol and Recurrent Events) trial, but only in one of 290 in the placebo group (P = .002).

"A recent study showed that 10 years of statin therapy increased women's risk of invasive ductal carcinoma by 83% and their risk of invasive lobular carcinoma of the breast by 97%."[92]

---

90 "Statins Do Not Protect Against Cancer: Quite the Opposite," Ravnskov et al, *Journal of Clinical Oncology*, online 20 January 2015, doi: 10.1200/JCO.2014.58.9564

91 Ravnskov U, Rosch PJ, McCully KS (2012) The statin-low cholesterol-cancer conundrum. QJM 105:383-388

92 McDougall JA, Malone KE, Daling JR, et al. (2013) Long-term statin use and risk of ductal and lobular breast cancer among women 55 to 74 years of age. *Cancer Epidemiol Biomarkers*

A study of the effects of simvastatin on 47,000 people found patients *tripled* their risk of dying from cancer within six years.[93]

Ravnskov and his team noted that while the statins themselves probably are not carcinogenic, their effectiveness at lowering so called 'bad' cholesterol probably is:

"This adverse effect results from their ability to lower blood lipids. More than a dozen research groups have documented that lipoproteins, particularly LDL, partake in the immune system by binding and inactivating all kinds of microorganisms and their toxic products. Because certain microorganisms have been incriminated as a possible cause of different malignancies, including colorectal cancer, it is difficult to understand how lowering LDL cholesterol could prevent cancer.

"Association never proves causation. Although it may be difficult to prove that statins can cause or prevent cancer, the preponderance of evidence favors the former."

You are going to hear screams from the establishment on this, but the evidence that low cholesterol causes cancer is strong, as a review published June 2016 makes clear:[94]

"Another explanation for an inverse association between LDL-C and mortality is that high cholesterol, and therefore high LDL-C, may protect against cancer. The reason may be that many cancer types are caused by viruses.

"Nine cohort studies including more than 140 000 individu-

Prev 22:1529-1537

93 Matsuzaki M, Kita T, Mabuchi H, et al. (2002) Large scale cohort study of the relationship between serum cholesterol concentration and coronary events with low-dose simvastatin therapy in Japanese patients with hypercholesterolemia. *Circ J* 66:1087-1095.

94 Ravnskov U, Diamond DM, Hama R, et al. "Lack of an association or an inverse association between low-density-lipoprotein cholesterol and mortality in the elderly: a systematic review". *BMJ Open* 2016;6: e010401. doi:10.1136/bmjopen-2015-010401

als followed for 10–30 years have found an inverse association between cancer and TC measured at the start of the study, even after excluding deaths that occurred during the first 4 years.

"Furthermore, cholesterol-lowering experiments on rodents have resulted in cancer, and in several case–control studies of patients with cancer and controls matched for age and sex, significantly more patients with cancer have been on cholesterol-lowering treatment.

"In agreement with these findings, cancer mortality is significantly lower in individuals with familial hypercholesterolaemia [high cholesterol]."

So what have we learned? That 'bad' LDL cholesterol may actually be crucial for helping your immune system to fight cancer, and that therefore the public health obsession with lowering cholesterol may fall into the category of 'be careful what you wish for'.

A New Zealand study has found public health messaging has whipped the citizens into line and delivered exactly what officials wished for. Serum (total) cholesterol of 9,000 people was measured across three surveys taken in 1989, 1997 and 2009.[95] The results showed the average "serum cholesterol decreased from 6.15 mmol/L in 1989 to 5.39 mmol/L in 2008/09. Mean saturated fat intake decreased from 15.9% of energy intake in 1989 to 13.1% in 2008/09. Between 1997 and 2008/09, unsaturated fat intake increased and fat from butter and milk decreased.

"Conclusions: The decrease in serum cholesterol is substantially

95 Miller, J. C., Smith, C., Williams, S. M., Mann, J. I., Brown, R. C., Parnell, W. R. and Skeaff, C. M. (2016), Trends in serum total cholesterol and dietary fat intakes in New Zealand between 1989 and 2009. *Australian and New Zealand Journal of Public Health*, 40: 263-269. doi: 10.1111/1753-6405.12504

larger than reported for many other high-income countries, and occurred in parallel with changes in dietary fat intakes and, for older adults, increased use of cholesterol-lowering medications.

"Implication: Given the demonstrated role of reduced saturated fat intake on lowering serum cholesterol, and as population average serum cholesterol levels and saturated fat intakes exceed recommended levels, initiatives to further encourage reductions in saturated fat are imperative."

A similar sort of one-track thinking dominated the sunsmart skin cancer messages promoted around the world—a dermatology-focussed approach to a minor killer (melanoma) led to widespread messaging to avoid the sun. Then scientists discovered the advice was dangerously reducing population levels of Vitamin D—essential for immunity, heart health and cancer prevention—which could be far more hazardous to health overall than the risk of melanoma.

It's all about balance, and a holistic approach to health rather than concentrating on an individual element so closely that you can't see the forest for the trees.

Which is exactly the point being made by researchers from the University of Auckland and AUT university, in response to the Otago University support for the establishment position on fats—the bottom line is not whether heart disease rates are improved, but whether lives are actually saved:[96]

"If saturated fat reduces CVD without adverse effects on other outcomes, we would expect overall mortality to be reduced.

---

96 "Chewing the saturated fat: should we or shouldn't we?", Thornley et al, *NZMJ* 23 May 2014, Vol 127 No 1394, pp 94-96

"Death is measured with less error than any other disease-specific outcomes. Focus on overall mortality avoids the risk of concluding that an intervention improves one endpoint, but, in reality, is offset by harm to another. For example, a treatment may reduce CVD but increase cancer incidence, so that the effect on overall mortality is neutral."

The Auckland team then listed some big studies, including the gold standard Cochrane Collaboration, which have failed to find any evidence that eating less fat saves lives. Surely, they pointed out, with so many people reducing their fat intake over recent decades and lowering cholesterol, we should have hard evidence by now.

"We ask ourselves, 'How much more evidence is needed before saturated-fat-based interventions are abandoned?' Popper stated that the hallmark of the scientific method is that a hypothesis is possible to falsify, should it lack supporting evidence.

"In the absence of a strong indication of harm, we believe the public should be left to chew the saturated fat, and concern themselves with avoiding dietary factors which consistently cause ill health."

Others are saying the same thing:

"Paradoxically, cholesterol lowering remains the focus of cardiovascular disease prevention despite the inconsistent benefit demonstrated in dozens of clinical trials. The cholesterol-lowering, statin-centric approach to cardiovascular disease prevention may in fact distract us from other beneficial therapies," says Robert DuBroff.

"Dr. Alexander Leaf, former chief of medicine at Massachusetts General Hospital, commented on this paradox and the Lyon Diet

Heart Study nearly 15 years ago by writing, 'At a time when health professionals, the pharmaceutical industries, and the research funding and regulatory agencies are almost totally focused on lowering plasma cholesterol levels by drugs, it is heartening to see a well-conducted study finding that relatively simple dietary changes achieved greater reductions in risk of all-cause and coronary heart disease mortality in a secondary prevention trial than any of the cholesterol-lowering studies to date' (Leaf, 1999)."[97]

Others say the whole 'kilojoule intake' approach to obesity is a failure, because it fails to take account of the fact that different foods can balance each other and deliver benefits greater than the sum of their ingredients:

"An energy-imbalance concept of obesity is oversimplified. Whereas short-term weight loss can be achieved by any type of calorie-reduced diet, in the long term, counting calories may not be biologically nor behaviorally relevant.

"Rather, the quality and types of foods consumed influence diverse pathways related to weight homeostasis, such as satiety, hunger, brain reward, glucose-insulin responses, hepatic de novo lipogenesis, adipocyte function, metabolic expenditure, and the microbiome. Thus, all calories are not equal...for the integrity of weight regulation."[98]

The benefits of the Mediterranean diet, say researchers, may not lie in specific areas like cholesterol or fats, but in the balance of the foods consumed—whole grains, salads, cheese,

---

97 "Does IMPROVE-IT prove it?", Robert DuBroff, *Preventive Medicine* Volume 85, April 2016, Pages 32-35 doi:10.1016/j.ypmed.2016.01.004
98 "Dietary and Policy Priorities for Cardiovascular Disease, Diabetes, and Obesity A Comprehensive Review Dariush Mozaffarian, *Circulation* Vol 133 Issue 2, http://dx.doi.org/10.1161/CIRCULATIONAHA.115.018585 Published: January 12, 2016

olive oil, lamb, poultry—which act together in different ways in synergy. Sodium's effect on blood pressure for example can be balanced by potassium intake—a banana.[99] In this way the negative effects of isolated ingredients are minimised while their positives help us stay healthy.

This is where research into what our ancestors ate—the so-called 'Paleo diet'—kicks in. There are three key ingredients to our meals: carbohydrates, fats and protein. Fooling around with the mix achieves different and surprising results.

"On an isocaloric basis, the diet with the highest protein and fat contents gives rise to the lowest weight gain," reported the *Journal of Nutritional Biochemistry* in 2016. Hi-fat, low-carbs, equals a better body.[100]

That study identifies what appears to be the 'heart' of the problem. LDL cholestrol levels *are* lowered by reducing saturated fat intake, but there are two kinds of LDL. Reducing animal fats reduces 'large particle' LDL, but it has no impact on 'small particle' LDL and it is the smaller particles that bind onto arterial walls. Even worse, it turns out dietary fats help keep the small particles under control, so by removing saturated fats we actually let lower LDL cholesterol levels do more damage.

Expressed in clinical terms for the doctors reading this:

"Since [the 1970s], dietary fat, and especially the consumption of SFA, has been consistently demonized. Yet, the reduction in LDL-C from reducing SFA intake seems to be specific for large and buoyant low-density lipoprotein (LDL) particles, while the small

---

99 *Transactions Of The American Clinical And Climatological Association*, VOL. 126, 2015 "Why Your Mother Was Right: How Potassium Intake Reduces Blood Pressure" by David H. Ellison
100 B. Ruiz-Núñez et al. / *Journal of Nutritional Biochemistry* 36 (2016) 1-20

and dense LDL particles are in fact the ones implicated in CVD. Accordingly, the levels of small dense LDL have been shown to increase in response to low-fat/high-CHO [carbohydrate] diets."

Delivering, arguably, a slap in the face to establishment cholesterol advocates, the study points out the lack of connection between eating fatty food and blood cholesterol levels: "SFA consumptions of 15% and 4% may correspond with TC [total cholesterol] values of 3 and 6 mmol/L, respectively, illustrating that SFA intake only explains a small part of TC variation."

In other words, someone eating four times as much saturated fat can have a cholesterol reading of three, yet a person basically avoiding SFA can have a cholesterol level double that. Yet what was it the University of Otago team said?

"Given the demonstrated role of reduced saturated fat intake on lowering serum cholesterol, and as population average serum cholesterol levels and saturated fat intakes exceed recommended levels, initiatives to further encourage reductions in saturated fat are imperative."

The Food Police are on the verge of determining what you are allowed to eat and how much extra sinful food tax you should pay, based on out of date science. Do you believe them?

Let's look at specifics. If, like me, you've bought into the low fat theme, you probably drink no-fat milk instead of whole milk. I've been that way for more than 20 years. So imagine my surprise to discover a University of Auckland study that found no difference in cholesterol or cardio health between low-fat and full-fat milk drinkers over six months, with one vital exception: those on *no*-fat milk *gained twice as much weight* over that time (800gm) as full-fat milk drinkers (400gm).[101] Go

---

101 "Effects of High and Low Fat Dairy Food on Cardio-Metabolic Risk Factors: A Meta-

figure. More proof, perhaps, that low fat diets cause obesity. I've gained weight on my low fat diet and I haven't touched butter in 30 years.

A recent study confirmed dairy fats may actually be protective for heart health.[102]

Then there's red meat. In 2010 a meta-analysis (pooling of multiple studies) found absolutely no connection between enjoying a steak and developing heart disease.[103] The perceived risks surrounding CVD and Type 2 diabetes were said to result from processed meats. A similar finding in regard to cancer was made in 2015:[104]

"In these two large cohorts of US health professionals, *processed* meat intake was positively associated with risk of Colo-Rectal Cancer, particularly distal cancer, with little evidence that higher intake of unprocessed red meat substantially increased risk of CRC."

In other words, avoid sausages, pies, burgers, cured meats and you will lower your risk. Eat high fibre foods (a balanced diet like mother recommended) and your risk will be further reduced.

In the WHO's Global Burden of Disease study, red meat ranked last in a list of 43 risk factors for disease.[105]

Analysis of Randomized Studies", Benatar et al, *PLoS ONE* 8(10):e76480 · October 2013, DOI: 10.1371/journal.pone.0076480

102 Qin Li-Qiang LQ. "Dairy consumption and risk of cardiovascular disease: an updated meta-analysis of prospective cohort studies". *Asia Pac J Clin Nutr* 2015; 24(3):90-100.

103 Micha R, Wallace S, Mozaffarian D. Red and processed meat consumption and risk of incident coronary heart disease, stroke, and diabetes mellitus: a systematic review and meta-analysis. *Circulation* 2010;121:2271-83.

104 "Processed and Unprocessed Red Meat and Risk of Colorectal Cancer: Analysis by Tumor Location and Modification by Time", Bernstein et al, *PLoS ONE* August 25, 2015 http://dx.doi.org/10.1371/journal.pone.0135959

105 "A comparative risk assessment of burden of disease and injury attributable to 67

As one expert pointed out, "the traditionally living Maasai, with intakes of both meat and milk that highly surpass the median Western (saturated) fat intake, present the highest [fat] content ever measured by our group, both in red blood cells and breast milk. They have an average TC of 4.9 mmol/L and almost no evidence of CVD."[106]

All of which is kind of echoed by another big study published July 2016 that supports the 'establishment' view of saturated fat.

Using data obtained from the American Health Professionals and Nurses studies, the team found that total dietary fat intake was protective against mortality, compared to those people who lowered fat and went hi-carb.[107]

"Intake of SFA, when substituted for total carbohydrates, was not significantly associated with CVD mortality."

The highest consumers of vegetable oils had the same cholesterol intakes as those consuming high levels of saturated fats, but had the best mortality risk.

The study did however find a link between saturated fats and death from respiratory illness—a 56% increased risk. It also states that replacing some saturated fats with vegetable oils can lower mortality.

However some of the most interesting news came on neurodegenerative disease mortality. All natural fats—saturated,

risk factors and risk factor clusters in 21 regions, 1990-2010: a systematic analysis for the Global Burden of Disease Study 2010 (vol 380, pg 2224, 2012)" Lim et al, *The Lancet* 381(9874):1276-1276 · April 2013

106 "The relation of saturated fatty acids with low-grade inflammation and cardiovascular disease," B. Ruiz-Núñez et al. / *Journal of Nutritional Biochemistry* 36 (2016) 1-20 http://dx.doi.org/10.1016/j.jnutbio.2015.12.007

107 Association of Specific Dietary Fats With Total and Cause-Specific Mortality," Wang et al, *JAMA Intern Med.* Published online July 05, 2016. doi:10.1001/jamainternmed.2016.2417

polyunsaturated and monounsaturated—were associated with a reduced risk of Alzheimer's, Parkinson's or the like. Omega 3 oils particularly so. However, trans-fatty acids used in processed foods, like hydrogenated vegetable oils and margarines, are associated with up to 66% increased risk of neurodegenerative death.

The take home message from this study, which its authors admitted was limited because it was observational rather than a trial, is again the need for a balanced diet and to eat fresh rather than processed food. Higher fat intake and lower carbs is associated with a healthier life, whereas the low-fat high carbs diet is associated with death. A diet with a mix of saturated and unsaturated fat is healthier overall.

The quality of carbohydrate is also important. Natural carbs from wholegrains and fresh food are healthy, but the majority of our carbohydrate intake comes from processed foods, refined sugars and alcohol, all of which raise mortality risk.

Another endorsement of paleo, perhaps.

In case you are wondering how to process the Wang study against the other big one on the Minnesota randomised trials, the key word is 'trial'. There are *observation* studies for Africa, like Wang et al, that appear to show benefits from vegetable oils. But every time there's a clinical *trial*—the gold standard in medical science—the apparent benefits of vegetable oils melt away.

As Ramsden said in the Sydney study:

"Advice to substitute polyunsaturated fats for saturated fats is a key component of worldwide dietary guidelines for coronary heart disease risk reduction. However, clinical benefits of the most abundant polyunsaturated fatty acid, omega 6 linoleic acid, have not been established.[108]

---

108 Ramsden CE, Zamora D, Leelarthaepin B, et al. Use of dietary linoleic acid for secondary

"In this cohort, substituting dietary linoleic acid in place of saturated fats increased the rates of death from all causes, coronary heart disease, and cardiovascular disease. An updated meta-analysis of linoleic acid intervention trials showed no evidence of cardiovascular benefit. These findings could have important implications for worldwide dietary advice to substitute omega 6 linoleic acid, or polyunsaturated fats in general, for saturated fats."

In other words, next time you hear a health official pushing the establishment line without solid clinical trial evidence, take it with a grain of salt (medicinal, of course).

There is one other point worth mentioning. Studies have drawn a distinction between trans-fats created during food processing (toxic) and trans-fats created naturally inside animals we eat. It appears the latter, predominantly known as CLAs, have health benefits:[109]

"CLAs have anticarcinogenic [anti-cancer], antiartherogenic [improving arteries], antidiabetic, and antiadipogenic [anti-obesity] properties (Geay and others 2001[110]; Khanal and Olson 2004[111]; Meľuchová and others 2008[112]). It has also been

prevention of coronary heart disease and death: evaluation of recovered data from the Sydney Diet Heart Study and updated meta-analysis. *BMJ* 2013;346:e8707. doi:10.1136/bmj. e8707

109 Howes, N. L., Bekhit, A. E.-D. A., Burritt, D. J. and Campbell, A. W. (2015), Opportunities and Implications of Pasture-Based Lamb Fattening to Enhance the Long-Chain Fatty Acid Composition in Meat. *Comprehensive Reviews in Food Science and Food Safety*, 14: 22–36. doi: 10.1111/1541-4337.12118

110 "Effect of nutritional factors on biochemical, structural and metabolic characteristics of muscles in ruminants, consequences on dietetic value and sensorial qualities of meat," Geay et al, *Reprod. Nutr. Dev.* 41 (2001) 1-26 DOI: 10.1051/rnd:2001108

111 "Factors Affecting Conjugated Linoleic Acid (CLA) Content in Milk, Meat, and Egg: A Review," R.C. Khanal and K.C. Olson, *Pakistan Journal of Nutrition:* 2004 | Volume: 3 | Issue: 2 | Page No.: 82-98 DOI: 10.3923/pjn.2004.82.98

112 "Seasonal variations in fatty acid composition of pasture forage plants and CLA content

claimed that high levels of CLA supplementation enhances muscle growth, but there are limited data supporting this claim (McGuire and McGuire 2000)."

In fact, so promising has the early research on natural trans-fats been that the meat industry is trying to figure out how to create even higher levels in cattle and sheep.

In 2015, de Souza reported a 42% risk reduction for diabetes when ruminant trans-fats were part of the diet.[113]

Animal fats (including natural trans-fats) good, omega-6 vegetable oils bad.

Chapter Summary
Main Points On Cholesterol

- low cholesterol policy dominates public health advice as a way to prevent heart disease
- researchers say current advice is based on flawed 1960s science
- clinical studies actually find people with low cholesterol are much more likely to die from heart disease
- clinical studies actually find people with low cholesterol are much more likely to develop cancer
- randomised controlled trials have shown no mortality benefit for people who lower their cholesterol by eating less saturated fat

---

in ewe milk fat", Meluchová et al, *Small Ruminant Research* August 2008 Volume 78, Issues 1-3, Pages 56-65 DOI: http://dx.doi.org/10.1016/j.smallrumres.2008.05.001
113 "Intake of saturated and trans unsaturated fatty acids and risk of all cause mortality, cardiovascular disease, and type 2 diabetes: systematic review and meta-analysis of observational studies," de Souza et al, *BMJ* 2015;351:h3978 doi: 10.1136/bmj.h3978

- the type of fat you eat (as long as you avoid industrial trans fats) has little impact on your blood cholesterol or mortality
- low cholesterol levels are associated with higher risk of death
- a balanced diet based primarily on unprocessed foods is more healthy than a low-fat diet
- high cholesterol may be largely irrelevant to your health

All of that said, let's look at natural health. We spend a fortune on supplements, but what is our diet adding to the mix, and do supplements actually work?

4

The Blurred Line Between Natural and Pharmaceutical

I F YOU'VE GOT this far you've probably guessed that modern medical science is in somewhat of a crisis and searching for answers behind the scenes. In one way, that's a good thing. True scientific advancement has nearly always come about as a result of ignoring tribalist principles like "consensus". Any academic who argues in any forum "the science is set-tled" without adding the cautionary words, "for now", doesn't deserve to wear the "scientist" badge. History has shown us time and again that settled science can be turned on its head by new discoveries, or realisations that previous calculations and theories are wrong.

In science, it boils down to two words: true or false. Something is true until it is proven false.

Back in the heyday of the 20th century, human civilisation jumped from horse and cart to landing on the moon in the space of a generation; from barely knowing what an atom was to unleashing the nuclear fury of a split atom on the world. In medicine, the discovery of antibiotics ushered in a new era of incredibly high confidence that doctors could find a cure for anything, and that a man-made pill was the answer.

To give medical science its due, some stunning gains have been made. We do live longer, because infections like a scratch on the arm that could once have almost certainly killed us have been controlled, "for now" (the issue of the post-antibiotic era will be canvassed later). That has meant attention has shifted from opportunistic infectious diseases to the so-called chronic diseases like cancer and heart failure, that appear to arise from lifestyle. And that's where medical researchers are sitting with their heads buried in their hands, because the science that seemed so clear 30 or 40 years ago is now looking distinctly "unsettled".

Pharmaceutical drug interventions have had limited success, and our efforts against cancer are largely blunt instrument chemotherapy where doctors wage nuclear war on tumours using the patient's body as the battleground. There's a strong element of 'cross your fingers and pray' in modern medicine, despite all of the trillions spent on healthcare globally over the years.

This is why there's been a blurring of the lines between pharmaceutical and natural. Pharmaceutical companies have always looked to nature for medical inspiration—the discovery of penicillin on mouldy bread is just one example—but they bring a different mindset: the belief that they can somehow isolate one ingredient that will make a difference, and patent it to make a fortune. In some cases they have, while in others they bang their heads against the wall as yet another new drug that looked great in lab tests fails to work in the real world.

Why is that?

Perhaps one of the answers can be found hidden in plain sight: synergy. For eons, humans have eaten meals comprised of a multitude of natural ingredients. Each meal can be expressed as a complex series of organic and inorganic chemicals and minerals, a symphony of elements that work together to nourish and fuel the body.

Plucking one chemical out of thousands and promoting it as the next big thing might be great for the balance sheet, but does it really do the job on its own or does it only work in combination with other chemicals?

Reading through the medical research literature, looking at how some of these clinical trials are done, you can be forgiven for the nagging suspicion that there's an awful lot of guesswork based on hypothesis involved, and that the end result is more like a game of pin the tail on the donkey.

Increasingly, researchers are beginning to think that nutrition and health is the sum of its parts, rather than isolated ingredients.

Take salt, for example. It can cause blood pressure to rise, but potassium can cause blood pressure to drop. Adding salt to a high potassium food like a baked potato could have an overall neutral effect, which could also explain studies finding it hard to blame salt for blood pressure: while we know the impact of sodium in isolation, no one has a diet that only consists of salt. They eat foods that could balance it. The meal works in synergy, not as isolated active ingredients. Studies looking at one ingredient may be missing the forest for the trees. Unless the study is sensitive to the complex interactions of dietary intakes, and more to the point the large variances from one person to another, its findings will be general.

As a result of all this, attention is now turning to a more holistic analysis, like determining what the myriad of ingredients in fresh unprocessed food might actually do. Are these chemicals the secret to better health?

To illustrate the point, researchers compiled a table setting out the different types of nutritional phytochemicals available in plants:

TABLE 1 [114]

Polyphenols

1. Flavonoids

Flavonols: quercetin, kaempferol (onions, kale, leeks, broccoli, buckwheat, red grapes, tea, apples)

Flavones: apigenin, luteolin (celery, herbs, parsley, chamomile, rooibos tea, capsicum pepper)

Isoflavones: genistein, daidzein, glycitein (soya, beans, chick peas, alfalfa, peanuts)

Flavanones: naringenin, hesperitin (citrus fruit)

Anthocyanidins (red grapes, blueberries, cherries, strawberries, blackberries, raspberries, tea)

---

114 Courtesy "Phytochemicals in cancer prevention and management?", Robert Thomas, Elizabeth Butler, Fabio Macchi and Madeleine Williams, *British Journal of Medical Practitioners*, June 2015, Volume 8, Number 2 http://www.pomi-t.com/Polyphenol-and-Cancer-Review.pdf. Table reprinted under Creative Commons Attribution-NonCommercial-NoDerivatives 4.0 International License

Flavan-3-ols (tannins): catechins, epicatechin, epigallocatechin gallate (tea, chocolate, grapes)
Flavanolols: silymarin, silibinin, aromadedrin (milk thistle, red onions)
Dihydrochalcones: phloridzin, aspalathin (apples, rooibos tea)

2. Phenolic acids

Hydrobenzoic acids: gallic acid, ellagic acid, vanillic acid (rhubarb, grape seed, raspberries, blackberries, pomegranate, vanilla, tea)
Hydroxycinnamic acids: ferulic acid, P-coumaric acid, caffeic acid, sinapic acid (wheat bran, cinnamon, coffee, kiwi fruit, plums, blueberries)

3. Other non-flavonoid polyphenols

Other tannins (cereals, fruits, berries, beans, nuts, wine, cocoa)
Curcuminoids: curcumin (turmeric)
Stilbenes: cinnamic acid, resveratrol (grapes, wine, blueberries, peanuts, raspberries)
Lignans: secoisolariciresinol, enterolactone, sesamin (grains, flaxseed, sesame seeds)

Terpenoids

1. Carotenoid terpenoids

Alpha, beta and gamma carotene (sweet potato, carrots, pumpkin, kale)

Lutein (corn, eggs, kale, spinach, red pepper, pumpkin, oranges, rhubarb, plum, mango, papaya)
Zeaxanthin (corn, eggs, kale, spinach, red pepper, pumpkin, oranges)
Lycopene (tomatoes, watermelon, pink grapefruit, guava, papaya)
Astaxanthin (salmon, shrimp, krill, crab)

2. Non-carotenoid terpenoids

Saponins (chickpeas, soya beans)
Limonene (the rind of citrus fruits)
Perillyl Alcohol (cherries, caraway seeds, mint)
Phytosterols: natural cholesterols, siosterol, stigmasterol, campesterol (vegetable oils, cereal grains, nuts, shoots, seeds and their oils, whole grains, legumes)
Ursolic acid (apples, cranberries, prunes, peppermint, oregano, thyme)
Ginkgolide and bilobalide (Ginkgo biloba)

Thiols

Glucosinolates: isothiocyanates (sulforaphane) and dithiolthiones (cruciferous vegetables such as broccoli, asparagus, brussel sprouts, cauliflower, horseradish, radish and mustard)
Allylic sulfides: allicin and S-allyl cysteine (garlic, leeks, onions)
Indoles: Indole-3-carbinol (broccoli, Brussel sprouts)

Other phytochemicals

Betaines found in beetroot
Chlorophylls found in green leafy vegetables
Capsaicin found in chilli
Peperine in black peppers

And that's just scratching the surface. As you'll discover in the next chapter, coffee on its own has a magnitude more chemicals than those listed here.

The point about these phytochemicals and antioxidants however is this: in lab tests, they have been shown to work with the immune system, reduce damage from ageing and fight cancer. But what do the studies show?

We've already examined three big areas of the Western diet—salt, chocolate and fats. Let's find out what happens with our most popular drinks. Could phytochemicals in coffee and tea save our lives?

5

The Beverages

Coffee

Humans have accessed sources of caffeine for a long time, but not directly from coffee beans until much later in the piece. It is found also in tea and cocoa, and it was these two plants we turned to first. The Chinese began harvesting tea around five thousand years ago, and we've already covered the origins of chocolate. It wasn't until the 1400s that the Arabs commercialised trade in the beans the world has come to know and love.

Coffee is, after water, the most popular daily drink in the USA with more than 400 million cups brewed there in any 24 hour period. As one study notes, if coffee is healthy or harmful, medical science needs to know.[115]

Coffee is what scientists call a "complex" food, comprising

115 "Effects of Habitual Coffee Consumption on Cardiometabolic Disease, Cardiovascular Health, and All-Cause Mortality," O'Keefe et al, *Journal of the American College of Cardiology* Vol. 62, No. 12, 2013
http://dx.doi.org/10.1016/j.jacc.2013.06.035

more than a *thousand* different chemicals. One of them—1,3,7-trimethylpurine-2,6-dione—is the molecule we prefer to call by the less intimidating name "caffeine". Other zingers in your flat white or latte include a "myriad bioactive substances with either health-promoting effects (e.g. chlorogenic acid, phenolic compounds and derived antioxidants, melanoidins, trigonelline-derived niacin) or potentially negative health effects (diterpene alcohols, acrylamide, 5-hydroxymethylfurfural metabolized into potentially harmful 5-sulfooxymethylfurfural)."[116]

The precise mix of angels and demons in the brew depends partly on how processed it is and also the brewing style (filter, espresso, instant).

With so many ingredients, the science on coffee hasn't fully come to the boil, which is why there are conflicting studies as researchers try and figure out just what coffee is capable of, but some things we do know.

Firstly, it is one heck of a stimulant—possibly one of the most widely used drugs on the planet. In addition to the tea and coffee consumed each day directly, food companies now inject caffeine or its clones into soft and energy drinks, alertness tablets and other products catering to those needs.

Secondly, coffee—like chocolate and fresh vegetables and fruit—is rich in antioxidants. This probably needs some explanation.

If you think of rust for a moment, technically that is oxidation—a breakdown of pure iron into iron oxide (rust) as a result of exposure to air and moisture. A similar process happens in living organisms. We rust, although we call it 'ageing'.

---

116 Caffeine and cardiovascular diseases: critical review of current research," Zulli et al, *Eur J Nutr*, Feb 2016, DOI 10.1007/s00394-016-1179-z

You may have heard the term 'free radicals'. These are molecules with an unbalanced electric charge. Atoms have a nucleus of positively charged protons, and orbiting that like planets are negatively charged electrons. The electrons orbit in pairs, but when they lose an electron through carelessness it creates a free radical. Those atoms that are in balance don't cause too much grief—they are stable. For those with an odd number of electrons, however, stability only comes by falling into the orbit of another out of balance atom or stealing an electron from somewhere.

In a way, this is a mini nuclear reaction. Atomic bombs work on the principle of throwing small amounts of unstable metal together (where hundreds of protons and electrons are ready to go haywire) so that they form a "critical mass" and explode. The reason radiation harms you is because a giant dose of free radicals tear through your body all at once leaving it unable to repair the damage.

So on a much smaller scale, free radicals in our daily lives are a form of radiation. Inside the body, those unstable electrons, atoms or molecules ferret around until they find something to bond with, and if it is one of your cells they reach stability with then they cause damage inside you—like cancer and degrading DNA.

Oxygen is one of those. We can't do without it, but it's volatile and unbalanced. Fires can't burn underwater because they can't access air—specifically the oxygen in the air. When a fire burns, it is actually oxidising, rusting with flare. The more oxygen, the more explosive it will get. In coal mine explosions it is not the build-up of methane gas that triggers the explosion—it is the mix of methane and oxygen hitting critical mass.

Oxygen inside your body is looking for a fight, it wants something to bind with.

Hence the term 'antioxidants'. These are compounds that bind to free radicals so they don't bind to you. If you have high circulating antioxidants, chances are they will act like little magnets to the free radicals—leaving you healthier and younger looking.

As you will have guessed, however, the war against getting older is a battle we are destined to lose from the moment we are born. We can delay a premature death by making good choices, but we cannot cheat death itself—eventually you will cash your ticket, and chances are it will be a non-infectious chronic disease that gets you.

"Non-communicable diseases, also known as chronic diseases (CDs), are adverse health conditions of long duration and generally, also of slow progression. The five main types of CDs are cardiovascular diseases, like heart attacks and stroke; cancer; chronic respiratory diseases, such as chronic obstructed pulmonary disease and asthma; diabetes; and neurodegenerative diseases, such as Parkinson's and Alzheimer's diseases. These CDs cause 63% of all deaths worldwide (36 million out 57 million global deaths)."[117]

Many of these diseases are incredibly hard to treat. Alzheimer's and Parkinson's for example are incurable, and it is only recently that scientists have discovered sunlight and Vitamin D can actually help reverse some Alzheimer's damage—something no drug has ever achieved.[118]

---

117 "Phenolic compounds in fruits and beverages consumed as part of the Mediterranean diet: their role in prevention of chronic diseases," Aguilera et al, *Phytochem Rev*, online 20 October 2015, DOI 10.1007/s11101-015-9443-z
118 *Vitamin D: Is This The Miracle Vitamin?* by Ian Wishart, Howling At The Moon, 2012, ISBN 9780987657312

Medical attention is increasingly turning to the natural world, to discover whether chronic disease is caused by our industrial lifestyles and therefore whether lifestyle and diet changes can boost our odds and deal us a better hand in the game of life.

Enter, coffee. A moment ago we talked about free radicals damaging DNA. One of the points they attack are telomeres, a string of DNA at the end of each chromosome in a cell which acts like protective covering on the ends of the chromosome. In a sense, telomeres prevent our chromosomes from unravelling or being damaged. The longer our telomeres are, the more youthful we are physically.

The problem in humans is that free radicals damage telomeres which in turn leaves our chromosomes vulnerable to ageing or cancer. However, the news is not all bad.

A recent study indicates your morning coffee may be an elixir of youth.

"No study, to our knowledge, has examined whether varying coffee or caffeine consumption levels are associated with telomere length, a biomarker of aging whose shortening can be accelerated by oxidative stress."[119]

To find out, researchers looked at the diets of a group of American women in the Nurses' Health Study, and examined blood samples to test telomere length.

"Higher total coffee consumption was significantly associated with longer telomeres after potential confounding adjustment. Compared with non-coffee drinkers, multivariable ORs for those drinking 2 to <3 and ≥3 cups of coffee/d were, respec-

---

119 Coffee Consumption Is Positively Associated with Longer Leukocyte Telomere Length in the Nurses' Health Study," Liu et al, *Journal of Nutrition*, June 8, 2016, doi: 10.3945/jn.116.230490

tively, 1.29 (95% CI: 0.99, 1.68) and 1.36 (95% CI: 1.04, 1.78) (P-trend = 0.02)."

Expressed in English, women who drank between two and three coffees a day were 1.29 times more likely (or 29% better odds ratio) to have longer telomeres, rising to 36% more likely if they consumed more than three cups daily. This is after taking into account variables like age and other factors.

"We found that higher coffee consumption is associated with longer telomeres among female nurses. Future studies are needed to better understand the influence of coffee consumption on telomeres, which may uncover new knowledge of how coffee consumption affects health and longevity."

They suspect it comes back to rich antioxidants that stop our cells from 'rusting':

"As example, a glass of red wine or a cup of tea or coffee contains about 100 mg polyphenols. Cereals, cocoa, and dry legumes also contribute to the polyphenol intake, being their total dietary intake about 1 g/day. Of nutritional interest, their levels are much higher than all other known dietary antioxidants, about tenfold than vitamin C and 100-fold than vitamin E and carotenoids."[120]

In 1991, researchers looked at a sample of 6,434 cognitively healthy Canadians in 1991 aged 65 or older. By cognitively healthy, none had developed signs of Alzheimer's or dementia at that point.

Five years later, the sample was checked again. Eighteen hundred of them had died within that five years, but of the

---

[120] Rodriguez-Mateos A, Vauzour D, Krueger CG et al (2014a) "Bioavailability, bioactivity and impact on health of dietary flavonoids and related compounds: an update." *Arch Toxicol* 88(10):1803-1853

4615 still alive, 194 were now diagnosed with Alzheimer's, and 3,894 were still classed as "cognitively normal".[121]

"Use of nonsteroidal anti-inflammatory drugs, wine consumption, coffee consumption, and regular physical activity were associated with a reduced risk of Alzheimer's disease. No statistically significant association was found for family history of dementia, sex, history of depression, estrogen replacement therapy, head trauma, antiperspirant or antacid use, smoking, high blood pressure, heart disease, or stroke."

Specifically, the reduced risk was large:

"Wine consumption reduced the risk by 50 percent. Other variables observed to be significantly associated with a lower risk of Alzheimer's disease were daily coffee consumption and regular physical activity (31 percent reductions for both). No association with tea drinking... was noted."

That last point is interesting, because tea also contains caffeine. Whatever the benefit from coffee, it must have been some other chemical.

A more recent study of 34,000 people published similar findings in 2016:[122] "Daily drinking of 1–2 cups of coffee was inversely linked with the occurrence of cognitive disorders (i.e., Alzheimer's disease, dementia, cognitive decline, and cognitive impairment), and the pooled RR (95% CI) was 0.82."

In other words, an 18% reduction in risk compared with those who drink coffee less frequently or not at all.

121 Lindsay J, Laurin D, Verreault R et al (2002) Risk factors for Alzheimer's disease: a prospective analysis from the Canadian study of health and aging. *Am J Epidemiol* 156(5):445-453 DOI: 10.1093/aje/kwf074

122 "Coffee intake and the incident risk of cognitive disorders: A dose-response meta-analysis of nine prospective cohort studies," Lei Wu et al, *Clinical Nutrition*, online 30 May 2016, doi:10.1016/j.clnu.2016.05.015

A study of 91,000 Japanese aged from 40-69 looked for a link between coffee drinking and mortality from the 'big three': cancer, cerebrovascular disease, or ischemic heart disease.

Over the next 19 years, nearly 13,000 of the sample died, but coffee was inversely linked to risk of death.[123]

"We showed an inverse association between coffee intake and total mortality in both men and women. HRs (95% CIs) for total death in subjects who consumed coffee compared with those who never drank coffee were 0.91 (0.86–0.95) for <1 cup/d, 0.85 (0.81–0.90) for 1–2 cups/d, 0.76 (0.70–0.83) for 3–4 cups/d, and 0.85 (0.75–0.98) for >5 cups/d (P-trend < 0.001). Coffee was inversely associated with mortality from heart disease, cerebrovascular disease, and respiratory disease.

"With this prospective study, we suggest that the habitual intake of coffee is associated with lower risk of total mortality and 3 leading causes of death in Japan."

Again, for those unused to reading Hazards Ratio (HR) reports, people who drank less than 1 cup a day had a 9% risk reduction, rising to 24% less risk of kicking up the daisies for people drinking three to four coffees a day. The smaller the P-trend number, incidentally, the more statistically significant the result.

Which of the 1000 bioavailable compounds is responsible? We don't know.

Melanoma, too, doesn't like it if you are a coffee lush. A study followed 447,000 white Americans for a decade, and found people who drank four cups or more of coffee cut their risks of malignant melanoma an average of 25%: "The highest

---

123 Association of coffee intake with total and cause-specific mortality in a Japanese population: the Japan Public Health Center-based Prospective Study," Saito et al, doi: 10.3945/ ajcn.114.104273 *Am J Clin Nutr* May 2015 *vol. 101 no. 5* 1029-1037

category of coffee intake was inversely associated with malignant melanoma," the study reported 2015. It had to be real
coffee—decaf didn't deliver the benefit.[124]

Another Japanese study has thrown up a contradiction however. It found that heavy coffee drinkers—more than five cups
a day—boosted their risk of a particular kind of brain bleed
known as a sub-arachnoid haemorrhage (SAR) by 279%. This
may sound spectacular, but only 304 people in the study drank
that amount of coffee, so it was not a big survey sample. Four
people suffered SAR—three women and one man. People taking
that much coffee also tended to be heavy drinkers and smokers,
so if they were a slot machine all three lemons were lighting up.[125]

A Swedish study of nearly 35,000 women over 11 years
revealed an instant drop in risk of stroke with the consumption of even one coffee a day, peaking at a 25% reduced risk
for 3-4 cups/d.[126] The benefits disappear and turn into a 20%
increased risk overall if you put sugar in the drink.[127]

Coffee has been shown to cause acute heart events and
stroke, but in people not used to coffee and who were given
high doses. Studies have found negligible effect on people with
a tolerance of caffeine. Coffee is safe for people recovering
from heart attacks.

---

124 "Coffee drinking and cutaneous melanoma risk in the NIH-AARP diet and health study,"
Loftfield et al, *J Natl Cancer Inst.* 2015 Jan 20;107(2). pii: dju421. doi: 10.1093/jnci/dju421.
Print 2015 Feb.
125 "Coffee Consumption and Incidence of Subarachnoid Hemorrhage: The Jichi Medical
School Cohort Study", Tsuyako Sakamaki, *J Epidemiol* 2016;26(2):71-75 doi:10.2188/jea.
JE20150092
126 Larsson SC, Virtamo J, Wolk A. Coffee consumption and risk of stroke in women. *Stroke*
2011;42:908-12.
127 "Sweetened Beverage Consumption Is Associated with Increased Risk of Stroke in
Women and Men," Larsson et al, *J. Nutr.* 2014;144:856-860

Caffeine, incidentally, is in a class of its own. It can rapidly increase your heart rate, cause a heightened mental state, and can cause "higher accessibility of dopamine, epinephrine, norepinephrine and serotonin"—mood enhancers. It is processed by the liver and hits the bloodstream in peak concentration within 30 to 120 minutes after consumption. With a half-life of 3-6 hours on average, plenty of caffeine can still be in your system long after your last cup of the day.

That, it turns out, can be a good thing. The metabolism of caffeine in the liver has a massive protective effect against liver cancer. One recent Italian study[128] found people who drank even just one cup of coffee a day slashed their risk of liver cancer by 40% compared with people who didn't drink coffee. People drinking three cups a day reduced the risk by 50%. The benefits persisted even for those who regularly drank alcohol—a known risk factor for liver cancer, which is ranked #3 on the world's deadliest cancers list.

Other cancers that coffee may help prevent include pancreatic, and specifically in women endometrial and colon cancer.

People who drink four coffees a day can reduce their risk of Type 2 diabetes by 28%.[129]

As the O'Keefe study concluded:[130]

---

128 Francesca Bravi, Cristina Bosetti, Alessandra Tavani, Silvano Gallus, Carlo La Vecchia. Coffee Reduces Risk for Hepatocellular Carcinoma: An Updated Meta-analysis. *Clinical Gastroenterology and Hepatology*, 2013; 11 (11): 1413 DOI: 10.1016/j.cgh.2013.04.039
129 van Dam RM, Hu FB. Coffee consumption and risk of type 2 diabetes: a systematic review. *JAMA* 2005;294:97-104. See also Huxley R, Lee CM, Barzi F, et al. Coffee, decaffeinated coffee, and tea consumption in relation to incident type 2 diabetes mellitus: a systematic review with meta-analysis. *Arch Intern Med* 2009;169:2053-63. doi:10.1001/archinternmed.2009.439
130 "Effects of Habitual Coffee Consumption on Cardiometabolic Disease, Cardiovascular Health, and All-Cause Mortality," O'Keefe et al, *Journal of the American College of Cardiology*

"Caffeine is a central nervous system stimulant, and its regular use typically causes mild physical dependence as evidenced by the development of tolerance, withdrawal symptoms (headaches, irritability, fatigue, depressed mood, anxiety, and difficulty concentrating), and cravings with abstinence.

"Notwithstanding, daily caffeine use generally does not threaten one's physical health and emotional/social well-being the way that many addictive drugs like alcohol, opiates, cocaine, and methamphetamines do; thus, substance abuse experts generally do not consider caffeine dependence a serious addiction. Indeed the tendency for coffee to promote habitual daily consumption may ultimately turn out to be advantageous if its myriad potential health benefits are confirmed.

"Caffeine, in moderate daily doses of 300 mg, or 3 cups of coffee, appears to be safe and harmless for healthy adults. Conversely, ingesting 10 times that amount of caffeine in a short period could be lethal. Moderation, tending toward 2 or 3 to as much as 4 cups a day if tolerated, seems a reasonable suggestion."

Tea

Not to be outdone by its muscular bean-derived rival, the more delicate teas of the world are also pulling their weight healthwise. Coffee may be the go-to poison for Westerners, but tea remains the most consumed drink globally. While green tea has always been seen as the cool kid of the family, ordinary tea is a heavy hitter in its own right. Both varieties are the same plant; the difference is that black tea is fermented during processing and green tea is not.

Vol. 62, No. 12, 2013 http://dx.doi.org/10.1016/j.jacc.2013.06.035

A fascinating study from Poland reveals that while the more 'natural' green tea has twice the level of antioxidants as fermented black tea, those in black tea are more water soluble (and thus bioavailable) than green tea, where experiments found a solution of ethyl acetate—an industrial solvent used in glue and nail polish—was the best way to extract the antioxidants.[131]

In practice then, black tea is more likely to deliver an effective dose of antioxidants, although that hasn't stopped researchers from extracting polyphenols into capsules:[132]

"Acute intervention studies using green tea polyphenols have shown protective effects against cancer. As example, green tea capsules (600 mg of flavan-3-ols/day) for 1 year resulted in only one tumor being diagnosed among the 30 subjects in the green tea group, versus 9 cancer diagnosed in the similarly sized control group (Bettuzzi et al. 2006[133]). Furthermore, consumption of five cups of green tea per day (400–500 mg of flavan-3-ols per cup) for 4 weeks on heavy smokers reduced the number of damaged cells by inducing cell growth arrest and apoptosis (Schwartz et al. 2005)."

In other words, green tea actually helped reverse the damage caused by smoking.

A Dutch study examined the diets and death rates of a sample of nearly 800 elderly men over 25 years. The researchers

131 Wojciechowski, Damian, Zbigniew Sroka, and Andrzej Gamian. "Investigation of antiradical potential of different kinds of teas and extracts from these teas using antiradical activity units (TAU)." Postepy Hig Med Dosw (online), 2011; 65: 796-803

132 "Phenolic compounds in fruits and beverages consumed as part of the Mediterranean diet: their role in prevention of chronic diseases," Aguilera et al, Phytochem Rev, online 20 October 2015, DOI 10.1007/s11101-015-9443-z

133 Bettuzzi S, Brausi M, Rizzi F et al (2006) Chemoprevention of human prostate cancer by oral administration of green tea catechins in volunteers with high-grade prostate intraepithelial neoplasia: a preliminary report from a one-year proof-of-principle study. Cancer Res 66(2):1234-1240

were looking at epicatechin, one of the tea antioxidants also found in chocolate.[134]

"The major dietary sources were tea (51%[of daily epicatechin intake]), apples (28%), and cocoa (7%). Risk of CHD [coronary heart disease] mortality was 38% lower in men in the top tertile of epicatechin intake than in men in the bottom tertile of epicatechin intake (HR: 0.62; 95% CI: 0.39, 0.98). Epicatechin intake was also significantly associated with 46% lower risk of CVD mortality in men with prevalent CVD (HR: 0.54; 95% CI: 0.31, 0.96) but not in men who were free of CVD.

"We show, for the first time to our knowledge, that epicatechin intake is inversely related to CHD mortality in elderly men and to CVD mortality in prevalent cases of CVD."

Apart from supporting the truism that "an apple a day keeps the doctor away", it also shows that ordinary tea packs an antioxidant punch.

A study of 164,000 Chinese men found that the 18% of the sample who drank green tea regularly reduced their CVD mortality risk by between 7-14%, and cancer mortality risk by between 14-21%.[135]

While drinking just one cup of coffee a day can slash your liver cancer risk by 40%, drinking the same amount of green tea has "no statistically significant association" according to a huge Asian study of 465,000 people.[136]

Another Asian study found green tea reduced risk of coro-

---

134 Dower, James I., et al. "Dietary epicatechin intake and 25-y risk of cardiovascular mortality: the Zutphen Elderly Study." *The American Journal of Clinical Nutrition* (2016): ajcn128819.
135 Liu, Junxiu, et al. "Association of green tea consumption with mortality from all-cause, cardiovascular disease and cancer in a Chinese cohort of 165,000 adult men." *European Journal of Epidemiology* (2016): 1-13.
136 Huang, Ya-Qing, et al. "Green tea and liver cancer risk: A meta-analysis of prospective cohort studies in Asian populations." *Nutrition* 32.1 (2016): 3-8.

nary heart disease by 11%, but with strings attached:[137]
"Interestingly, the above-mentioned association between green tea consumption and reduced risk of CHD incidence appeared to be more pronounced in individuals who were male, more than 60 years old, overweight or with diabetes," reported the study. It speculated that green tea may help with weightloss, thus being of benefit to men at high risk of CHD, whereas in women it decreases estrogen levels, and as estrogen protects women that could explain the lack of a coronary benefit for women—particularly post-menopause when estrogen production ceases and women's health problems increase.

Black tea, incidentally, is commonly and successfully used in high concentrations to terminate pregnancies in Africa,[138] so if you are trying to get pregnant, keep that risk in mind. One Canadian study found pregnant tea drinkers more than doubled their risk of developing pre-eclampsia, warning:

"Persistent tea drinking during pregnancy may be associated with an increased risk of pre-eclampsia."[139]

But it turns out the catechins in tea—whilst they may fight free radicals—could harm your unborn child. A Chinese study discovered the catechins interfere with folic acid levels, and tea drinking was associated with triple the risk of a baby born with neural tube defects:[140]

137 "Green tea consumption is associated with reduced incident CHD and improved CHD-related biomarkers in the Dongfeng-Tongji cohort," Chong Tian et al, *Sci Rep.* 2016; 6: 24353. Published online 2016 Apr 13. doi: 10.1038/srep24353
138 "Abortion experiences among Zanzibari women: a chain-referral sampling study," Norris et al, *Reproductive Health* 2016 13:23 DOI: 10.1186/s12978-016-0129-9
139 Wei, Shu-Qin, et al. "Tea consumption during pregnancy and the risk of pre-eclampsia." *International Journal of Gynecology & Obstetrics* 105.2 (2009): 123-126.
140 "Tea Drinking as a Risk Factor for Neural Tube Defects in Northern China," Ye et al, *Epidemiology* 2011;22: 491–496, DOI: 10.1097/EDE.0b013e31821b4526

"The elevated risk associated with daily tea drinking remained after adjusting for maternal age, educational level, occupation, and periconceptional folic acid supplementation. The association was present for all 3 major subtypes of NTDs (ie, anencephaly, spina bifida, and encephalocele)."

It appears that because tea affects enzymes that normally process folate, simply consuming more folate does not get around the problem—it's like pouring more water into a bucket with holes in the bottom.

"In healthy male volunteers, green and black tea, effectively reduced serum folate concentrations. Pregnant Japanese women who drank 4 or more cups of green tea per day were more likely to have a low serum folate concentration," warned the study.

Another study found women who drank one cup of green or black tea a day were twice as likely to suffer a spina bifida pregnancy, with the odds rising to a 180% increased risk at three or more cups a day.[141]

Conversely, another Chinese study found folate levels are not affected by tea.[142] It did, however, admit that much of its sample came from areas where cheaper teas with low levels of catechins were popular—meaning a less potent brew.

Some research links coffee to neural tube defects as well—possibly for the same reasons.[143] Another study found a 30%

---

141 "Prenatal tea consumption and risks of anencephaly and spina bifida," Correa et al, *Annals of Epidemiology* 10(7):476-477 · November 2000 DOI: 10.1016/S1047-2797(00)00144-7 · Source: PubMed

142 "Tea consumption is not associated with reduced plasma folate concentration among Chinese pregnant women," Liu et al Birth Defects Research Part A *Clinical and Molecular Teratology* 103(9) · June 2015 DOI: 10.1002/bdra.23398 · Source: PubMed

143 "Coffee-Induced Neural Tube Defects," Carlomagno et al, 2015 *Coffee in Health and*

increased risk of miscarriage from just one small latte a day, rising to a 120% increased risk with higher coffee intake: "The ingestion of caffeine may increase the risk of an early spontaneous abortion among non-smoking women."[144]

The advice with both of these globally popular beverages is to tread carefully if pregnant.

While some studies have found no benefit from tea on neuro-cognitive disorders (NCD), others have found the opposite. A longevity study of 957 elderly ethnic Chinese in Singapore over seven years found green tea drinkers cut their risk of senility by 57%, and black tea drinkers by 47%:[145]

"Reduced NCD risk was observed for both green tea (OR=0.43) and black/oolong tea (OR=0.53) and appeared to be influenced by the changing of tea consumption habit at follow-up. Using consistent non-tea consumers as the reference, only consistent tea consumers had reduced risk of NCD (OR=0.39). Stratified analyses indicated that tea consumption was associated with reduced risk of NCD among females (OR=0.32) and APOE ε4 carriers (OR=0.14) but not males and non APOE."

So women could enjoy up to 68% reduced risk of NCD, just by regularly drinking tea.

The flipside of teas—green or black—is that they are often grown in areas with high natural fluoride. Scientific testing

Disease Prevention, http://dx.doi.org/10.1016/B978-0-12-409517-5.00049-8

144 "Caffeine Intake and the Risk of First-Trimester Spontaneous Abortion," Cnattingius et al, *N Engl J Med 2000*; 343:1839-1845December 21, 2000DOI: 10.1056/NEJM200012213432503

145 "TEA consumption reduces the incidence of neurocognitive disorders: Findings from the Singapore Longitudinal Aging Study," L. Feng, *The Journal of Nutrition*, Health & Aging pp 1-8 First online: 15 January 2016

has shown average fluoride levels of two parts per million in an ordinary cup of tea. Decaffeinated teas approach 4.5ppm.[146] To put that in perspective, there is no established safe dose for fluoride, and toxic impact on IQ has been shown at intakes in fluoridated water above 1.5ppm[147]. Five cups of tea a day could give you anywhere from 12% to 300% of what health authorities call an "acceptable intake" of fluoride. And the official "acceptable" level is much higher than safety studies recommend.

Fluoride in coffee, on the other hand, is almost negligible, ranging from 0.1ppm to 0.6ppm.[148]

The take home message is that your antioxidant serving from green or black tea comes with baggage: heavy tea consumption gives you a fluoride dose like swallowing toothpaste.

Next: do fish oils really work?

---

146 "Tea fluoride concentration and the pediatric patient," Quock et al, *Food Chemistry* Volume 130, Issue 3, 1 February 2012, Pages 615-617, doi:10.1016/j.foodchem.2011.07.084
147 "Effect of fluoride exposure on the intelligence of school children", Saxena et al, *J Neurosci Rural Pract.* 2012 May-Aug; 3(2): 144-149. doi: 10.4103/0976-3147.98213, http://www.ncbi.nlm.nih.gov/pmc/articles/PMC3409983/
148 Warren, Donna P., Harold A. Henson, and Jarvis T. Chan. "Comparison of fluoride content in caffeinated, decaffeinated and instant coffee." *Fluoride* 29 (1996): 147-150.

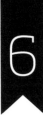

The Hunt For The Silver Bullets: Omega 3 vs Omega 6

I N THE PREVIOUS chapters, we've seen how foods we've been told to avoid are actually good for us in moderation, as part of a balanced diet, overturning half a century's worth of health messaging.

Our industrial diets, and increasing reliance on packaged or processed foods, have left us vulnerable to ingestion of food processing chemicals like dangerous trans fats[149], or with gaps in our nutrient levels.

One of the things that emerged from studies of the Mediterranean diet was the balance between omega-3 poly-

---

149 Ironically it is man-made industrial trans-fats that kill, while studies have shown that natural trans-fats like those found in animal meat may confer some slight protection Howes, N. L., Bekhit, A. E.-D. A., Burritt, D. J. and Campbell, A. W. (2015), Opportunities and Implications of Pasture-Based Lamb Fattening to Enhance the Long-Chain Fatty Acid Composition in Meat. Comprehensive Reviews in Food Science and Food Safety, 14: 22-36. doi: 10.1111/1541-4337.12118

unsaturated fatty acids (n3 PUFAs) and omega-6 (n6 PUFAs). The former come mostly from oily fish (and some plants) while the latter come primarily from grains and vegetable oils. Omega-6 oils can cause inflammation which can trigger chronic diseases. Although we need n6 oils, they need to be balanced with n3 oils.

Studies of the Inuit people in the arctic revealed lower rates of heart disease, high intake of omega-3s and low intake of omega-6—for the obvious reason that crops and vegetable oils were scarce in the arctic.

In a major review of the science on omega-3s, researchers set out how scientists back in 1971 were initially convinced that they held the key:[150]

"Interest in the cardioprotective effects of long chain omega-3 polyunsaturated fatty acids (LCn3) was largely influenced by the low rates of cardiovascular disease (CVD) amongst the Inuits of Greenland who consumed a high marine fat diet rich in LCn3s[151]. This finding stimulated years of epidemiological and clinical studies investigating the cardioprotective effects of LCn3s."

It was believed that omega-3s countered inflammation within the body and eased "pro-inflammatory effects of metabolic stress precipitated by poor diet and lifestyle."

What that statement doesn't address is vitamin D. The Inuit had high levels of vitamin D from oily fish and game meats like reindeer and seals. But back in 1971 we only thought vita-

---

150 "Controversies in omega-3 efficacy and novel concepts for application," Radcliffe et al, *Journal of Nutrition & Intermediary Metabolism* 5 (2016) 11-22, http://dx.doi.org/10.1016/j.jnim.2016.05.002

151 Bang HO, Dyerberg J, Nielsen AB. Plasma lipid and lipoprotein pattern in Greenlandic West-coast Eskimos. *Lancet* 1971;1(7710):1143e5.

min D was for bone health. It is only in the last decade that studies have shown a massive reduction in heart disease rates and cancers as well.

So the presumption of omega-3 researchers was that omega-3 was the silver bullet in the Inuit diet, and they've now spent decades trying to prove it, with mixed results:

"Although the original hypothesis of the link between LCn3s and CVD protection was based on a high LCn3 containing diet (namely a high marine fat diet) the majority of clinical trials since have focussed on EPA and DHA supplementation, and results of repeated meta-analyses have not shown conclusive evidence in support of their beneficial health effects."

When they use the word 'supplementation' they mean dietary supplements, not omega-3s in their natural state as part of a meal. So what they are saying is that having seen that the Inuit 'diet' was good, they tried to use supplements to get the same results, and failed. The importance of this will become clear shortly.

DHA, or docosahexaenoic acid, is found in fatty fish like salmon and sardines, along with EPA (eicosapentaenoic acid). Both oils are found in most omega-3 fish oil supplements, but they do different things. EPA has been found to lower very high triglyceride levels in the blood, but DPA has been found to increase levels of so-called 'bad' LDL cholesterol. However, DPA is essential for the brain. Do you see how complex this task of sorting out benefits is?

"Interestingly, the Inuit—regular fish-eaters—demonstrated the lowest CVD risk despite a high prevalence of obesity and smoking," noted a 2004 study.[152]

---

152 Ruxton CHS, Reed, Simpson MJA, et al. (2004) The health benefits of omega-3

Researchers have identified "blue zones"—areas of the planet where people often live beyond 100. Okinawa in Japan, Sardinia in the Mediterranean and a few others. There's one thing they all have in common—high levels of fish in the diet, and a reliance on some other key ingredients we've been learning about:

"Cardioprotective dietary patterns such as a Mediterranean style diet or a 'blue zones' type eating pattern include a wide variety of plant foods consumed with high levels of antioxidants and other bioactive nutrients that may act in a protective and synergistic way, increasing the quality of fatty acids incorporated into tissues."

Now, recall a moment ago how diet was good but supplements not so much? Here's another study:

"In the evidence published since 2007, this summary of evidence concludes that dietary intake of fish was found to be mostly consistent with respect to protection from heart disease and stroke. Higher fish intake was associated with lower incident rates of heart failure in addition to lower sudden cardiac death, stroke and myocardial infarction.[153]"

In 2004, scientists came up with a new criteria for assessing heart risk. They called it the "omega-3 index", and worked out through a math equation you risk. An index figure of 4% was "low cardioprotection", while a figure of 8% was "high cardioprotection":[154]

polyunsaturated fatty acids: a review of the evidence. *J Hum Nutr Diet* 17, 449-459.

153 *Heart, Lung and Circulation* Volume 24, Issue 8, August 2015, Pages 769-779 doi:10.1016/j.hlc.2015.03.020 "Indications for Omega-3 Long Chain Polyunsaturated Fatty Acid in the Prevention and Treatment of Cardiovascular Disease," Paul Nestel

154 doi: 10.1194/jlr.R027904 December 2012 *The Journal of Lipid Research*, 53, 2525-2545.

"For example, the average omega-3 index in Western countries is ~ 5% and the incidence of Sudden Cardiac Death is 150/100,000 person-years. In Japan, a country with a high fish consumption, the omega-3 index is greater than 9% and the incidence of SCD is 7.8/100,000 person-years in the general population."

Never mind the index, look at the heart attack rates there: Western 150/100,000py, Japan 8/100,000py.

Great. We eat fish, we are healthier. How does that translate to fish oil supplements?

"In relation to omega-3 LCPUFA supplementation, neither a beneficial nor adverse effect was demonstrated in primary or secondary prevention of coronary heart disease (CHD). Although the evidence continues to be positive for the role of omega-3 LCPUFA in the treatment of hypertriglyceridaemia [excessively high triglycerides] and a modest positive benefit in heart failure. No further evidence was found to support the consumption of 2 g alpha-linolenic acid (ALA [flaxseed oil])/day over the current Australian guidelines for 1 g/day."

Fascinating. Not just because the questionmarks continue over how to best deliver fish oil (in a pan or in a pill?), but also because flaxseed oil, the plant version of omega-3, was less than inspiring.

A small randomised trial at an Australian hospital tested a group of coronary patients. Half were fed a daily dose of fresh salmon, the other half took a fish oil tablet. In both groups the omega-3 levels went up, but those dining on fish got slimmer and enjoyed other benefits:[155]

---

155 BRAZIONIS, L., TING, E., ITSIOPOULOS, C., WILSON, A. and HODGE, A. (2012), The effects

"A decrease in blood pressure (>5 mmHg; P < 0.05) was observed after the fish but not the fish oil. The change in waist to hip ratio also favoured the fish intervention. Resting heart rate fell by a similar amount on both interventions, and the omega-3 index increased significantly on both; from 6% to 7–8% (P < 0.01). Blood lipids did not improve on either arm [of the trial]."

Another area where fish oil comes into its own is dementia. There is no drug treatment for Alzheimer's, and no way of stopping it once it has started—at least that was the case up until recently. Vitamin D at high doses was found to repair some of the damage and slow the progression of the disease.

That led science to experiment with natural remedies, and a recent Swiss review of the evidence comes down in favour of vitamins and fish oil:[156]

"One factor evidently important for neuronal health and function is the optimal supply of nutrients necessary for maintaining normal functioning of the brain. Mechanistic studies, epidemiologic analyses, and randomized controlled intervention trials provide insight to the positive effects of docosahexaenoic acid (DHA) and micronutrients such as the vitamin B family, and vitamins E, C, and D, in helping neurons to cope with aging.

"These nutrients are inexpensive in use, have virtually no side effects when used at recommended doses, are essential for life, have established modes of action, and are broadly accepted by

---

of fish or fish oil on the omega-3 index. *Nutrition & Dietetics,* 69: 5-12. doi: 10.1111/j.1747-0080.2011.01566.x

156 "Inadequate supply of vitamins and DHA in the elderly: Implications for brain aging and Alzheimer-type dementia", Mohajeri et al, *Nutrition,* February 2015 Volume 31, Issue 2, Pages 261-275, http://dx.doi.org/10.1016/j.nut.2014.06.016

the general public. This review provides some evidence that the use of vitamins and DHA for the aging population in general, and for individuals at risk in particular, is a viable alternative approach to delaying brain aging and for protecting against the onset of AD pathology."

More to the point, given that drugs don't work, natural remedies are the only tool in the box when it comes to keeping our brains sharp.

A randomised double blind trial of DHA fish oil on 485 Americans aged over 55 found 24 weeks of taking a supplement boosted verbal recognition memory in formal tests, but not working memory or executive function.[157]

Another trial, however, has found fish oil supplements are too weak to overwhelm Alzheimer's once it is underway. The clinical study of 295 patients in America on 2g of DHA a day found no difference between those on the fish oil and those given a placebo: the march of Alzheimer's over 18 months was relentless, leading the trial team to sadly note: "Supplementation with DHA compared with placebo did not slow the rate of cognitive and functional decline in patients with mild to moderate Alzheimer disease."[158]

Given the apparent contradiction between some trials that worked and some that did not, one analyst speculated that oxidisation of the oils themselves may be to blame:

"A possible theory behind the conflicting and lack of positive

---

157 "Beneficial effects of docosahexaenoic acid on cognition in age-related cognitive decline", Karin Yurko-Mauro et al, *Alzheimer's & Dementia* November 2010 Volume 6, Issue 6, Pages 456-464, http://dx.doi.org/10.1016/j.jalz.2010.01.013
158 "Docosahexaenoic Acid Supplementation and Cognitive Decline in Alzheimer Disease: A Randomized Trial," Quinn et al, *JAMA*. 2010;304(17):1903-1911. doi:10.1001/jama.2010.1510

results of supplement trials is the oxidisable nature of fish oil supplements which may reduce the bioavailability."[159]

That could also explain, putting aside the possible influence of vitamin D for a moment, the difference between those who eat fresh fish and those who take supplements.

"The question remains," says the Radcliffe review, "is it more than the LCn3 content of fish that has a role to play in both the secondary and primary prevention of disease? Are other nutrients present in fish important, or are dietary patterns associated with a high fish intake higher in other protective nutrients as well?"

Those other nutrients also include astaxanthin, selenium and the energy drink component taurine.

An exploration of the Mediterranean diet reveals frequent consumption of nuts—hazelnuts, almonds and walnuts primarily—which are sources of plant based omega-3 (a variety known as alpha linolenic acid or ALA). Not all omega-3s are created equal, however, as only around 8% of ALA converts to the EPA form in the body, and as little as 0.1% to DHA.[160]

This conversion process is more significant than you might think. Grass-fed beef (like New Zealand's for example) has five times the level of bioavailable omega-3s that grain-fed beef has.[161] This is because cattle naturally eat plants containing ALA, which they convert to EPA and DHA. So when we eat that beef, we get the benefit of pre-converted omega-3s.

---

159 Radcliffe et al, supra

160 "Long-chain n−3 PUFA: plant v. marine sources," Christine M. Williams, *Proceedings of the Nutrition Society* / Volume 65 / Issue 01 / February 2006, pp 42-50 DOI: http://dx.doi.org/10.1079/PNS2005473

161 Daley et al. A review of fatty acid profiles and antioxidant content in grass-fed and grain-fed beef. *Nutr J* 2010;9:1e12.

When we eat grain-fed beef, we don't. And when a scientific study reports on red meat, have they first checked whether it is grass-fed? Grass-fed red meat is actually a health food. It contains higher levels of B vitamins, beta carotene (converted to vitamin A in the body) and the antioxidant tocopherol (vitamin E). It contains lower levels of two saturated fats that can raise LDL cholesterol (although the issue surrounding cholesterol is now less clear cut than it seemed ten years ago).

The point is, however, that dietary sources of red meat can be key providers of omega-3 PUFAs, particularly as we eat it more often than fish:

"Although red meat cannot be compared to oily fish in terms of its actual LCn-3 PUFA content and overall fatty acid profile, it is possible that red meat makes a greater contribution to total dietary intakes of LCn-3 PUFA than oily fish based on the present levels of consumption," reported a British study.[162]

"This contention has been supported by Australian data, where the consumption of beef and lamb from predominantly grass-fed animals contributes 28% of total LCn-3 PUFA intakes, compared with 48% from oily fish."

It turns out that grass-fed mammals have another LCn3 that fish don't have, but which is also found in the fatty blubber of seals and marine mammals. It's known as DPA, not to be confused with fish oil DHA. It appears we can convert DPA to EPA when we eat it, so we turn animal fats into healthy omega-3s.

So, it figures that if you have cut grass-fed red meat out of

---

162 Red meat from animals offered a grass diet increases plasma and platelet n-3 PUFA in healthy consumers McAfee et al, *British Journal of Nutrition* (2011), 105, 80–89 doi:10.1017/ S0007114510003090

your diet, you may not be getting enough fresh omega-3s. This issue of freshness is important, and we will return to it soon.

In fact, that 2006 study from Australia went even further. By the time you added in steak pies, pork and poultry, "almost half the average adult intake of LCn3PUFA appears to originate from meat sources."[163]

Despite all that, scientists say we are still not getting enough:[164]

"Only 20% of the population meets the recommended n-3 LCPUFA intakes and only 10% of women of childbearing age meet the recommended docosahexaenoic acid (DHA) intake. Fish and seafood is by far the richest source of n-3 LCPUFA including DHA," reported an Australian review in 2016.

To illustrate the health potential of grass-fed meat, a British randomised double blind controlled trial fed one group of cattle and lambs on grass, and another group exclusively on grain for six weeks. At the end of that time the beasts were processed and fed in the trial to forty healthy volunteers in 100gm servings three times a week for four weeks, whose blood levels were taken at the start and again at the end.

Those who ate grass-fed meat saw their long chain omega-3 blood levels rise 35%, while those who ate grain-fed meat saw their LCn3 levels plummet by nearly the same amount.

Significantly, there was no impact on serum cholesterol levels at all in either group of meat-eaters despite an increase in saturated

---

163 "Dietary intake of long-chain omega-3 polyunsaturated fatty acids: contribution of meat sources," Howe et al, *Nutrition.* 2006 Jan;22(1):47-53. DOI:10.1016/j.nut.2005.05.009

164 "Australians are not Meeting the Recommended Intakes for Omega-3 Long Chain Polyunsaturated Fatty Acids: Results of an Analysis from the 2011-2012 National Nutrition and Physical Activity Survey," Meyer BJ. *Nutrients.* 2016 Feb 24;8(3):111. doi: 10.3390/nu8030111.

fat levels, which again goes to prove the point of the cholesterol chapter earlier and is great news for paleo followers and New Zealand and Australian grass-fed beef and lamb producers:[165]

"It is important to acknowledge the aspect that red meat consumption had no effect on serum cholesterol, TAG or blood pressure in the present study, as it concurs with other studies showing moderate red meat consumption has no negative effects to health.

"Overall, the results of the present study suggest that consumption of red meat from grass-fed animals may provide valuable amounts of LCn-3 PUFA to the consumer and increased production of red meat from grass-fed animals may thereby help to increase LCn-3 PUFA intakes of consumers."

And again, why are omega-3s important?

We know that they do reduce inflammation in our bodies, which can lead to cancer and heart disease among others. Omega-6 oils increase inflammation. But we also know of large cohort studies linking fish consumption to a longer life. For reasons already outlined, "fish" contain a number of healthy ingredients including the monster of modern research—vitamin D, so it is important when reading fish studies not to necessarily assume that it is just omega-3s at play.

The Nurses' Health Study from the 1980s, which is mentioned in earlier chapters, revealed that American women who ate fish (canned tuna, salmon, fresh fish, shrimp etc) five times a week or more reduced their risk of fatal heart disease by up to 45%.[166] Similar benefits exist for men.

165 McAfee et al, supra
166 "Fish and Omega-3 Fatty Acid Intake and Risk of Coronary Heart Disease in Women," Hu et al, *JAMA.* 2002;287(14):1815-1821. doi:10.1001/jama.287.14.1815.

A randomised controlled trial of omega-3 fish oil supplements holds what could be a major key. Known as the GISSI Trial from Italy, more than 11,000 patients who had recently survived a heart attack were assigned either fish oils, vitamin E or a placebo. What stunned researchers was that those on 1g/day fish oil had a big drop in mortality—a 45% reduction in sudden heart attack deaths.[167]

Yet this lifesaving change came without any lowering of cholesterol levels. Whatever omega-3 oils were doing, the cholesterol was irrelevant. This spooked the doctors who had been trained to believe that high cholesterol meant death and low cholesterol meant life. Here was a supplement they had expected to lower cholesterol—it hadn't. Yet it was saving lives regardless.

They needed to know how. It turned out other vegetable oils—the polyunsaturated fats scientists had urged us to increase in place of animal fats—were to blame for the heart attacks because omega-6 oils (arachidonic acid or 'AA') can cause heartbeats to trip up (arrhythmia).

"A not commonly known, but additional example relevant to this discussion," Alexander Leaf points out in an editorial in the journal *Circulation*,[168] "is that all the prostaglandins we tested (except prostacyclin) produced from AA are proarrhythmic, whereas the equivalent prostaglandins derived from EPA are not.

---

167 Marchioli R, Barzi F, Bomba E, et al, on behalf of the GISSI-Prevenzione Investigators. Early protection against sudden death by n-3 polyunsaturated fatty acids after myocardial infarction: time-course analysis of the results of the Gruppo Italiano per lo Studio della Sopravvivenza nell'Infarto Miocardico (GISSI)-Prevenzione. *Circulation*. 2002; 105: 1897-1903

168 On the Reanalysis of the GISSI-Prevenzione, Alexander Leaf, *Circulation* http://dx.doi.org/10.1161/01.CIR.0000015344.46176.99 Published: April 23, 2002

"The discussion in the preceding paragraph was to make the point that n-6 AA, when in excess in the diet and in our bodies, unbalanced by n-3 EPA+DHA may increase coronary atherosclerosis and sudden cardiac arrhythmic deaths."

So in plain English, when you cook your food in polyunsaturated vegetable oils or spread margarine, you are ingesting poison. More so than animal fats according to many studies. At the moment, our diets are so overloaded in omega-6 PUFAs that serum tests are showing ratios as high as 20:1 for n-6 vs. n-3 in our blood.[169]

"The optimal ratio," says Alexander Leaf, "appears to be closer to 1/1, which has been roughly estimated to be the ratio during the 2 million or so years when our hunter-gather forebears were adapting their genes to their environment including their diet.[170]"

That's because our paleo ancestors were not squeezing cooking oil out of omega-6 sunflower seeds, they were cooking in animal fats high in omega-3s and eating fish high in omega-3s.

When the GISSI team reanalysed their data, they found what had happened. Firstly, taking vitamin E didn't save anyone's life. Secondly, they found the omega-3 fish oils were delivering a benefit because of the olive oil used in cooking by the Italians. Olive oil is 77% monounsaturated oleic acid, but while the control group on placebos were also using olive oil, it wasn't changing the balance of n-6/n-3, and that was the key. Olive oil was neutral, so neutral plus omega-6 still equals omega-6.

---

169 Simopoulos A. Evolutionary aspects of diet and essential fatty acids. In: Hamazaki T, Okuyama H, eds. *Fatty Acids and Lipids: New Findings*. Basel, Switzerland: Karger; 2001: 18-27.
170 ibid

Whereas omega-3 plus neutral into an existing omega-6 diet lowered the n-6:n-3 ratio.

"To obtain maximal cardiovascular benefit from intake of n-3 PUFAs, it seems the concomitant intake of n-6 PUFAs must be reduced and n-3 PUFAs increased," writes Leaf.

Adding omega-3s from fish and red meat to your diet balances the ratio between omega-6 and omega-3. Olive oil doesn't perform miracles because it is olive oil—it performs miracles because it is *not* omega-6 polyunsaturated vegetable oil.

A recent study underscored just how much of a rat poison polyunsaturated vegetable oils are at the levels they appear in our diets, particularly in fast and processed food but even in smoothies and cereals if you are digesting omega-6 grains and seeds:[171]

"Omega-6 (n-6) and omega-3 (n-3) fatty acids are metabolically diverse with different physiological functions (Simopoulos 2002).

"Omega-3 fatty acids are important for regulating immune responses (Simopoulos 2002), aiding brain and vision development in fetuses, maintaining neural and visual tissues, and have recently been linked to reduced cancer, type-2 diabetes, and CVD (Benatti and others 2004).

"However, n-6 fatty acids, which account for most PUFAs in Western diets (Simopoulos 2002), are thought to have roles in the development of many diseases, including coronary heart disease, major depression, aging, and cancer, which are all distinguished by elevated levels of interleukin 1 (IL-1), levels

---

171 Howes, N. L., Bekhit, A. E.-D. A., Burritt, D. J. and Campbell, A. W. (2015), Opportunities and Implications of Pasture-Based Lamb Fattening to Enhance the Long-Chain Fatty Acid Composition in Meat. *Comprehensive Reviews in Food Science and Food Safety*, 14: 22-36. doi: 10.1111/1541-4337.12118

of which can be increased by elevated levels of n-6 fatty acids (Simopoulos 2002, 2008).

"Simultaneous increases in dietary n-3 and reductions in n-6 fatty acids lowers the n-6:n-3 ratio and has been shown to reduce CVD mortalities by up to 70% (Simopoulos 2008). Consequently, it has been suggested that the n-6:n-3 ratio should be below 4.0 in a healthy diet (Simopoulos 2004)."

So what cooking oils should you avoid like the plague?

TYPE	n-6	n-3	Harmful saturated fat (palmitic or myristic)
Rice bran oil	34.4%	2.2%	22.1%
Sunflower	39.8%	0.2%	5%
Peanut	33.4%	–	10%
Sesame	41%	–	8%
Safflower	75%	–	5%
Soybean	57.7%	–	10%
Palm	9.1%	–	44.5%
Corn	58%	1%	9%

A number of those oils are used in the food industry. You can see how high the n-6:n-3 ratios are within each oil. The missing balance of each oil percentage, incidentally, is mainly oleic acid (the main ingredient in olive oil), but it's a neutral backdrop to the omega-6 overload.

Which brings us back to fish oil supplements. The reality is that they work to reduce heart disease—not by lowering cholesterol but because they strike a balance with omega-6 intake and that neutralises most of the poison associated with omega-6.

Why not cut out omega-6 entirely? Because strangely we need certain levels of it for growth, reproduction and a host of other bodily requirements, yet thanks to 50 years of dietary advice to consume more PUFAs and omega-6 cereals and grains we are swimming in omega-6 and it is killing us. Telling us not to eat meat (which contains omega-3s) only made the imbalance even worse.

To illustrate the point another way, water is essential to life but if you drink too much in a short space of time you will in fact 'drown' from over-saturation. It's the same with omega 6. In the rush to avoid animal fats (needlessly in all likelihood), we turned to omega-6 and bumped our levels up unsafely. Now we are reaping the results of that 'health' fad.

But what about if everyone on the planet turns to fish oil? Well, if that happens the effect will be the same as if everyone buys an electric car and plugs it into the grid each night to charge. Collapse.

The world is already being overfished in the wild. Scientists have only discovered in the past decade that fish play a key role—like forests—in absorbing and processing CO_2[172]. The clearfelling of massive forests, and driftnetting of the oceans, are each having a huge impact on earth's ability to regulate CO_2—arguably a much bigger impact than humanity's actual carbon emissions.[173]

---

172 "Fishdunnit! Mystery solved", University of Miami news release, based on a study published in *Science*, 16 January 2009, http://www.rsmas.miami.edu/pressreleases/20090116-flounder.html

173 Human caused emissions account for about 3% of the total CO2 in circulation any given year. All of the CO2 is normally processed through natural sources and actual 'outgassing' can vary by 10 or 20% a year, but if you damage 30% of the planet's 'lungs', while concentrating on the much smaller 3% emissions, you are utterly missing the real problem. If the lungs worked fine the extra emissions wouldn't matter. The political ploy seems to be that it is easier to tax emissions and make the public feel guilty, than it is to reclaim land to replant

With one study pointing out it takes 3kg of seafood to grow a 2kg farmed fish, it looks as though mass fish-farming to meet demand for fish-oils could be unsustainable.[174] But there is one avenue of research: fish produce omega-3 by eating the omega-6 in marine plants like phytoplankton. They are more efficient at converting omega-6 to EPA and DHA than mammals are for the most part.

Scientists are now looking at modifying the gene sequence in cattle to make them more efficient at producing omega-3s.[175] That, of course, is a whole new debate for a different book, and it may not surprise you to learn that pesticide company Monsanto, DuPont and other giants are rushing to market with genetically engineered omega-3 products like Soyamega™ and Newharvest-EPA™.

An experiment in the lab with human breast cancer cells found that cells modified to produce omega-3s killed tumour cells, "whereas the control cancer cells with a high n-6/n-3 ratio continued to proliferate."[176] Proof, if you still needed it, that those nice polyunsaturated vegetable oils swirling through your system are not your friend, no matter how much government dieticians try to convince you otherwise.

Earlier in this chapter however you'll recall test results from fish oil supplements, as opposed to a diet of fish, were not

---

forests, and stop big multinational corporations from taking all the fish.

174 Leaf, 2002, supra

175 Kang ZB, Ge Y, Chen Z, et al. Adenoviral transfer of Caenorhabditis elegans n-3 fatty acid desaturase optimizes fatty acid composition in mammalian heart cells. *Proc Natl Acad Sci U S A.* 2001; 98: 4050-4054.

176 Ge Y-L, Chen Z, Kang ZB, et al. Effects of adenoviral transfer of Caenorhabditis elegans n-3 fatty acid desaturase on the lipid profile and growth of human breast cancer cells. *Anticancer Res.* 2002;22: 537-544.

always glowing. For some reason, the magic bullet of omega-3 pills didn't always work:[177]

"The UK Diet and Reinfarction Trial (DART) study showed that dietary advice to eat 2 portions of oily fish/wk decreased total mortality over the following 2 y by 29%. However, a second study (DART-2) by the same group, which used fish-oil supplements instead of fish in patients with stable angina, found no benefit and a trend for a less favourable [code for 'heart attack'] outcome in the supplemented group."

Or, as another researcher described it: "cardiac deaths and Sudden Cardiac Death increased significantly by 28% and 53%, respectively."[178]

We've since found out that it's not just about taking fish oil capsules, it's also about slashing your intake of omega-6 across the board as well. But there's something else: oxidation. Rust. Just like everything else, fish oils are vulnerable to free radicals. They lose potency quickly which is why you don't want them stored in your cupboard for too long, not much longer than you'd want to keep a fish in your cupboard in fact.

A study out of the University of Auckland's Liggins Institute drew hisses and growls from supplement makers after testing 32 brands of fish oil on sale in New Zealand and finding them below standard:

"Only 3 of 32 fish oil supplements contained quantities of

---

177 "Plant compared with marine n-3 fatty acid effects on cardiovascular risk factors and outcomes: what is the verdict?," Thomas AB Sanders doi: 10.3945/ajcn.113.071555 *Am J Clin Nutr* July 2014 vol. 100 no. Supplement 1 453S-458S

178 "Omega-3 fatty acid supplementation and cardiovascular disease: Thematic Review Series: New Lipid and Lipoprotein Targets for the Treatment of Cardiometabolic Diseases," Donald B. Jump et al December 2012 *The Journal of Lipid Research*, 53, 2525-2545. doi: 10.1194/jlr.R027904

eicosapentaenoic acid (EPA) and docosahexaenoic acid (DHA) that were equal or higher than labelled content, with most products tested (69%) containing <67%."

Ouch! If you can't trust the dose on the label, does that mean studies that found no benefits were compromised because the actual dose was too low?

Worse than that though—most of the fish oils had allegedly gone off inside their capsules.

"The vast majority of supplements exceeded recommended levels of oxidation markers. 83% products exceeded the recommended Peroxide Value levels, 25% exceeded AV [aldehydes and ketones] thresholds, and 50% exceeded recommended Totox [total allowable oxidation] levels. Only 8% met the international recommendations, not exceeding any of these indices.

"Almost all fish oil supplements available in the New Zealand market contain concentrations of EPA and DHA considerably lower than claimed by labels. Importantly, the majority of supplements tested exceeded the recommended indices of oxidative markers. Surprisingly, best-before date, cost, country of origin, and exclusivity were all poor markers of supplement quality."

Naturally, this study went down like a warm fish milkshake in the natural health industry around the world, especially as the study didn't name any brands.

One of New Zealand's leading suppliers, About Health, manufacturer of the "Lester's Oil" formulation of fish oil and vitamin D, arranged for an independent science lab to sniff its armpits just in case its products were fishy:

"Firstly, the researchers never named any brands, we think because they were unsure of the accuracy of their results, which means the whole industry is tarred by this dodgy research,"

CEO Dan King explained in a media statement." Therefore, there is no evidence that Lester's Oil or any other brands were involved. Regardless, I decided to 'take a bottle off the shelf' (metaphorically…we don't have shelves, we have dark boxes instead)

"We sent the bottle to AsureQuality; a leading, certified, independent lab in NZ and tested for total Omega-3 fatty acids—we advertise more than 500mg per capsule… the result came back as 535mg per capsule, this indicates extremely good quality, no degradation of note, and exceeding the label claim.

"The study at Auckland University is in my opinion, dodgy. It was not carried out by experts, and Dr. Laurence Eyres (the expert *Consumer Magazine* used to consult with for its market testing (in 2007), and Chairman of the Oil and Fats Association) stated that there are many things that can go wrong with these tests, they really need to be done by experts using validated methods and being part of proficiency testing programs."

Eyres was the consultant scientist for About Health, but his criticisms of methodology were backed up at a conference of supplement makers in Australia, where independent scientists confirmed they were not happy with the methodology either.

King quoted from some correspondence with a UK fish oil manufacturer, who suspected the samples had been thawed out too quickly:

"Our initial thoughts on this study are that the samples have been mishandled in some way during the analysis for both the oxidative parameters and the fatty acid profile to be so far removed from that claimed by the manufacturers. The other option is adulteration in some way during the processing however that seems extremely unlikely given so many samples have been affected. We have read the analytical preparation section and it seems to that there are some immediate differences in sample preparation. We also note that they have frozen samples at -80°C prior to analysis but no explanation as to how these have then been thawed for analysis. The warming up of the samples may well have contributed to this.

"Further it is known that peroxide values decrease over time as the primary oxidation products further decompose to secondary oxidative products (as recognised in the paper). The high PV and AV results seen in this report would indicate the oxidation is "fresh" rather than a long term degradation. The presence of a low AV coupled with a high PV would also indicate sample mishandling as if the product was badly oxidised then in reality you would expect this to be the other way round as oxidation is auto-catalytic."

The Auckland University study results were trumpeted by media around the world as proof that vitamins and supplements are little more than bottled cobra juice. The *New York Times* was scathing. But in the light of the media coverage, Australia's Therapeutic Goods Agency swooped on fish oils to test for themselves. They found no issues. The Australian government science agency the CSIRO had also done its own testing and found fish oils compliant with standards.

About Health, meanwhile, was particularly annoyed at the controversy's impact on public perception, especially as its own formulation had passed a clinical test with flying colours:[179]

"The supplement (Lester's Oil) was effective in improving

---

[179] The effects of a Vitamin D, Omega 3, Co-enzyme Q10, Zeaxanthin, Lutein and Astaxanthin supplement (Lester's Oil) on Healthy people. Part One: Effects on Inflammatory markers and Lipids." Laing et al, 2014

key inflammatory markers (CRP, HDL and Triglycerides) in healthy people."

Ironically, that study had also been done by Auckland University, which found it gave a 59% boost in omega-3 blood levels after four weeks—something unlikely if it had oxidised or been under strength.

Supplement manufacturers are still seething over the Albert et al study, accusing pharma giants of using it to defame natural supplements so they can gain market share for their genetically-modified versions.

A major scientific review of the omega-3 controversy said flawed or not, the study revealed a weakness in that scientists had been using over the counter supplements for clinical trials without double checking the quality for themselves:[180]

"The findings of the Albert et al. (2015) study have been disputed by experts at a recent scientific meeting, due to non-standard analysis techniques. Alternatively, other studies investigating disparity between product claimed concentrations of fatty acids and independent analysis showed similar concentrations between the manufacturer and independent analysis.

"Whilst analytical methodologies used should be validated and recognised, it is apparent that reliance on label reported EPA and DHA values weakens the strength of evidence from LCn3 supplement intervention studies. In the potential instance that previous studies with no effect from LCn3 intervention used a supplement that contained much lower quantities of LCn3 than indicated by manufacturer labelling, this may have affected outcomes of the study. This supports that future LCn3

---

180 Radcliffe et al, 2016, supra

supplementation studies should have independent analytical verification, using validated methods, of capsule fatty acid concentration."

But the controversy hasn't ended. Auckland University's Liggins Institute launched from the frying pan into the fire with a follow-up study in 2016, feeding oxidised fish oil to pregnant rats.[181] Their logic was that if most fish oils on the market were rancid, and pregnant women were taking them to boost their unborn baby's brain health, what might the effects be of eating a fish oil that had gone off.

Not content with common or garden-variety levels of 'offness', they ensured their test oils were rancid by baking them under a fluorescent light (generating UV radiation) and bubbling pure oxygen through them for 30 days, just like you would do at home. Then, instead of feeding the pregnant rats the equivalent of the 2g/day that a pregnant woman would take, they fed these rats the equivalent of 40 mls (three tablespoons) of rancid oil.

Then they expressed "surprise" when 30% of the newborn rat pups born to mothers on this dosage died.

"We were surprised by the death rate," said study lead Professor Wayne Cutfield, in a news release from the Liggins Institute. "We'd expected some negative health effects on the rat offspring, but we didn't expect them to die."[182]

"We don't know exactly why the newborn rats died," Dr Ben Albert from the Liggins team added. "Because we didn't expect them to die, we didn't design the study to look for reasons."

---

181 "Oxidised fish oil in rat pregnancy causes high newborn mortality and increases maternal insulin resistance", Albert et al, *American Journal of Physiology*–Regulatory, Integrative and Comparative Physiology Published 6 July 2016 Vol. no. , DOI: 10.1152/ajpregu.00005.2016
182 https://www.scimex.org/newsfeed/third-of-newborn-rats-died-if-mums-ate-bad-fish-oil

The study looked at three things: rats fed rancid fish oil, rats fed fresh fish oil, and the differences if either group was eating a high saturated fat diet[183] or alternatively a low fat diet. It was this diet test that actually produced some dynamite results.

Interestingly, and missed in all the media coverage, was this: newborn rats on oxidised fish oil died at a rate eight times higher than those in the control group fed a an ideal low fat/ high carb diet, but newborn rats whose mothers were fed fresh fish oil with a high saturated fat diet had an even lower death rate than the control group, which means fresh fish oil in association with a high fat diet actually reduced natural death rates.

Compared to rats eating a so-called ideal diet, three percent of whose newborn pups died, mothers on fish oils and lard reduced their risk of infant mortality by more than 60%. Only 1% of their pups died.

As a test between low fat and high fat diets...apparently a high saturated fat diet is healthier for you.

Naturally this inconvenient truth was overlooked in the media coverage. Equally naturally, other scientists were not impressed at the Liggins Institute study:[184]

"I was very concerned about the original paper, which they continually cite, and claim shows that most over the counter omega-3 supplements in New Zealand are oxidised," the Cancer Society's Professor Lynette Ferguson told the NZ Science Media Centre. "This conflicts with the data from the omega-3 centre in Australia.

---

183 http://www.researchdiets.com/opensource-diets/stock-diets/dio-series-diets see Diet 12451
184 www.sciencemediacentre.co.nz/2016/07/22/newborn-rats-died-after-mothers-fed-rancid-fish-oil-expert-reaction/

"Having done analytical work with these compounds myself, I am only too conscious that there are some technical difficulties in getting accurate results.

"The original problems are compounded by this paper. It uses oxidised oil that has had oxygen bubbled through it for 30 days plus light exposure.

"This is far beyond the level of contamination their earlier paper suggested was present in any New Zealand supplement. This oil was fed to animals at concentrations way beyond those appropriate to humans.

"If you look at their data, there was actually a minor benefit shown from the un-oxidised oil, suggesting a benefit to pregnant women of supplementation."

Dr Peter Nicholls, a senior research scientist with Australia's CSIRO, echoed the concerns:

"The wider scientific community was surprised and highly disappointed by the original 2015 *Scientific Reports* paper from University of Auckland researchers. The Australian Therapeutic Goods Administration (TGA) performed follow-up analyses and all tested oils were not oxidised and omega-3 content met label claims.

"For this new study, the justification appears to be driven by the *Scientific Reports* paper, which remains in the strongest doubt and dispute. The new paper uses heavily oxidised oil that the New Zealand authors prepared. As Australian and New Zealand fish oils are not heavily oxidised, the study is seen as not relevant," he told the SMC.

So, the take-home points so far from this chapter: we need omega-6 oils and omega-3 oils at a ratio of roughly one to one instead of currently 15 or 20 to one. Our diets are currently so overloaded in omega-6 oils that it is causing inflammation, type-2 diabetes, heart disease and cancer. A juicy steak, ironically, is a near perfect balance between its omega-6 and omega-3 content. This may be one reason why diabetes patients on paleo diets are reporting improvements in their health.

Omega-3 oils from fish and red meat are more bioavailable and effective than omega-3 plant oils like flaxseed. Red meat, pork and poultry actually provide nearly half of our current (inadequate) omega-3 intake.

Most of our margarines and oils used in commercial food processing are omega-6 dominant PUFAs and New Zealand's Ministry of Health, just by way of example, is *still* urging people to use PUFAs despite the growing evidence that it kills:

"Reducing saturated fat intake and partially replacing it with unsaturated fats, in particular polyunsaturated fats, is linked with a decreased risk of cardiovascular disease[185]... Choose and/ or prepare foods and drinks: with unsaturated fats (canola, olive, rice bran or vegetable oil, or margarine) instead of saturated fats (butter, cream, lard, dripping, coconut oil)."[186]

They get points for mentioning olive oil but not for rice bran, vegetable oil or margarine. And of course, we've seen how omega-6 PUFAs can cause heart attacks, not decrease them. Just another example of health authorities dishing out potentially deadly advice.

Why are health authorities saying this? The answer is simple: omega-6 PUFAs lower cholesterol, which is why all those margarines made by the big chemical companies are pushing

185 http://www.health.govt.nz/system/files/documents/publications/eag-summary.pdf
186 http://www.health.govt.nz/system/files/documents/publications/eating-activity-guidelines-for-new-zealand-adults-oct15_0.pdf

themselves as "proven to lower cholesterol". Well yes, it does, and we've seen studies in the Cholesterol chapter proving that you are more likely to die prematurely with low cholesterol. That's not stopping the big guns of the American Heart Association from pushing the mantra:[187]

"The replacement of 10% of calories from saturated fatty acid with omega-6 PUFA is associated with an 18-mg/dL decrease in LDL cholesterol, greater than that observed with similar replacement with carbohydrate. These findings confirm an LDL-lowering effect of omega-6 PUFA beyond that produced by the removal of saturated fatty acids. Favourable effects of LA on cholesterol levels are thus well documented and would predict significant reductions in CHD risk."

Except as we now know, they don't reduce Coronary Heart Disease risk. The cholesterol debate is increasingly looking like an 'Emperor's New Clothes' parable, and if low cholesterol is actually a killer as the studies are now showing, then anything giving you low cholesterol—like omega-6 polyunsaturated vegetable oils and margarines—could be helping you to save the deposit for your own little patch of land at Pleasant Meadows Lawn Cemetery. The pharmaceutical giants sell you the food that makes you sick, then sell the medicines to treat your illness. They will make a fortune off you in the twilight of your life as your health fails. Everyone wins. Except you.

It would be fair to say that the matter of whether omega-6 is

---

187 "Omega-6 Fatty Acids and Risk for Cardiovascular Disease: A Science Advisory From the American Heart Association Nutrition Subcommittee of the Council on Nutrition, Physical Activity, and Metabolism; Council on Cardiovascular Nursing; and Council on Epidemiology and Prevention," Harris et al, *Circulation* Feb 2009 http://dx.doi.org/10.1161/CIRCULATIONAHA.108.191627

safe or toxic to us in high doses (remembering that some intake of omega-6 is essential) remains hotly debated, and the empire is continually striking back with public assurances, including a claim that the omega ratio does not matter:

"Existing evidence suggests beneficial effect of dietary linoleic acid for cardiovascular outcomes, not harm, and use of the ratio of n-6 to n-3 is unlikely to impart meaningful information over and above assessment of the individual fatty acids alone," stated a group of scientists in 2015. The review carried a conflict of interest disclosure, however:[188]

"Disclosures: Dr Mozaffarian reports ad hoc travel reimbursement or honoraria from Bunge, Pollock Institute, Quaker Oats, and Life Sciences Research Organization; ad hoc consulting fees from McKinsey Health Systems Institute, Foodminds, Nutrition Impact, Amarin, Omthera, and Winston and Strawn LLP; membership on the Unilever North America Scientific Advisory Board; royalties from UpToDate; and research grants from the National Institutes of Health. The other authors report no conflicts."

However, a Japanese study on heart patients found those with the best n3:n6 ratio had a 50% drop in major adverse cardiac events, so the claim that the ratio is irrelevant appears to be wrong.[189] Another Japanese study found those with the highest omega-6 levels and the worst ratio were 83% more likely to develop coro-

---

188 Response to Letters Regarding Article, "Circulating Omega-6 Polyunsaturated Fatty Acids and Total and Cause-Specific Mortality: The Cardiovascular Health Study", *Circulation*, (Circulation. 2015;132:e25-e26. DOI: 10.1161/CIRCULATIONAHA.115.014853.
189 "Ischemic Heart Disease: Ratio of Serum n-3 to n-6 Polyunsaturated Fatty Acids and the Incidence of Major Adverse Cardiac Events in Patients Undergoing Percutaneous Coronary Intervention," Domei et al, *Circulation Journal* Vol. 76 (2012) No. 2 p. 423-429 http://doi.org/10.1253/circj.CJ-11-0941

nary lesions. The study noted "Eicosapentaenoic acid (EPA) of the omega-3 polyunsaturated fatty acids (n-3 PUFA) family plays important roles in the prevention of cardiovascular disease (CVD), while, arachidonic acid (AA) of the n-6 PUFA family promotes inflammatory and prothrombotic influences."[190]

Heart patients admitted to hospital were also found much more likely to have coronary plaque if they had a high omega-6 to omega-3 ratio.

"A low serum EPA level and a low EPA/AA ratio was associated with high vulnerability of coronary plaques."[191]

You are twice as likely to die—that's the blunt warning from a 2015 study of heart failure patients based on their omega-6 ratios: "Cardiac mortality was significantly higher in the low EPA/AA group than in the high EPA/AA group (12.7 vs. 5.9%, log-rank P = .004)... The EPA/AA ratio was an independent predictor of cardiac mortality in patients with HF; therefore, the prognosis of patients with HF may be improved by taking appropriate management to control the EPA/AA balance."[192]

These were not associative studies based on diet questionnaires—these were angiograms and blood tests on actual heart patients that revealed not only their PUFA ratio but also the heart damage they were sustaining.

Patients on kidney dialysis are also much more likely to

190 "Association of Plasma Omega-3 to Omega-6 Polyunsaturated Fatty Acid Ratio with Complexity of Coronary Artery Lesion," Hayakawa et al, *Internal Medicine* Vol. 51 (2012) No. 9 P 1009-1014 http://doi.org/10.2169/internalmedicine.51.7162
191 "Relationship Between Coronary Plaque Vulnerability and Serum n-3/n-6 Polyunsaturated Fatty Acid Ratio," Kashiyama et al, *Circulation Journal* Vol. 75 (2011) No. 10 p. 2432-2438 http://doi.org/10.1253/circj.CJ-11-0352
192 Watanabe, Shunsuke, et al. "Associations With Eicosapentaenoic Acid to Arachidonic Acid Ratio and Mortality in Hospitalized Heart Failure Patients." *Journal of Cardiac Failure* (2016). doi:10.1016/j.cardfail.2016.04.017

develop heart disease if they have a high omega-6 ratio (low EPA):[193]

"These data suggest that low ratios of both EPA/AA ratio and n-3/n-6 PUFAs were closely associated with carotid atherosclerosis in patients on Haemodialysis."

Health bureaucrats keep saying 'ignore the ratio, there's nothing to see here', but in real clinical situations it can literally be the difference between life and death.

The well-regarded Cochrane Collaboration reviewed omega-6 randomised controlled trials, in light of the controversy, and in 2016 stated it couldn't decide if polyunsaturated fats were good or bad:[194] "There is a need for larger well conducted RCTs assessing cardiovascular events as well as cardiovascular risk factors."

In other words, it is way too early to be issuing assurances that omega-6 oils and margarines are safe—let alone promoting them as 'good for the heart' as some margarine manufacturers like Unilever are doing.

As a major review recently concluded: "Ideally, reverting the n-3:n-6 PUFAs ratio in human diet back to the original 1:1 rather than the current 1:15 should lessen the incidence of chronic-degenerative diseases."[195]

Another scientific review is equally blunt:[196]

---

193 Umemoto, Norio, et al. "Reverse association of omega-3/omega-6 polyunsaturated fatty acids ratios with carotid atherosclerosis in patients on hemodialysis." *Atherosclerosis* 249 (2016): 65-69.

194 Al Khudairy, Lena, et al. "Omega 6 fatty acids for the primary prevention of cardiovascular disease." *The Cochrane Library* (2015).

195 A review of recent evidence in human studies of n-3 and n-6 PUFA intake on cardiovascular disease, cancer, and depressive disorders: does the ratio really matter?," Marventanoa et al, *International Journal of Food Sciences and Nutrition* Volume 66, Issue 6, 2015 pages 611-622 DOI: 10.3109/09637486.2015.1077790

196 "Evolutionary Aspects of the Dietary Omega-6/Omega-3 Fatty Acid Ratio: Medical

"Excessive amounts of n-6 polyunsaturated fatty acids (PUFAs) and a very high n-6/n-3 ratio, as is found in today's Western diets, promote the pathogenesis of many diseases including cardiovascular disease, cancer, and inflammatory and autoimmune diseases. On the contrary, increased levels of n-3 PUFA (a lower n-6/n-3 ratio) exert suppressive effects. We thus recommend that n-3 and n-6 fatty acids should be distinguished on food labels because they both are metabolically and functionally distinct and have opposing physiological effects. We further argue that a lower ratio of n-6/n-3 fatty acids is desirable as it is likely to reduce the risk of many of the chronic diseases of high prevalence in Western societies, as well as in the developing countries."

Because of ethics restrictions, doctors are not allowed to knowingly test suspected toxins on humans even though direct intervention is the best experimental science of all. They can, however, experiment on hamsters. In light of the American Heart Association's global assurance that omega-6 oils and margarines are good for you, researchers decided to test that theory on animals. Thank God they did.

One set of hamsters was allowed to live the high life with a diet of saturated animal fats—lashings of lard like your rotund old uncle used to sit down to (the same one the rats were fed).

Another group were placed on a low-fat/high carb diet, and the third group were fed omega-6 polyunsaturated fats. A control group of hamsters eating an ordinary hamster diet were allowed to watch.[197]

Implications," Artemis P. Simopoulos, *Evolutionary Thinking in Medicine: Part of the series Advances in the Evolutionary Analysis of Human Behaviour* pp 119-134 Date: 14 May 2016
197 "High intake of saturated fat, but not polyunsaturated fat, improves survival in heart failure despite persistent mitochondrial defects," Galvao et al, *Cardiovascular Research,*

The BMI of both sets of hamsters getting extra fats increased 10% over the study.

The *first* hamsters to pop their clogs were the omega-6 team. Fully half of their number were dead by day 260 of the experiment. Fifty percent of the low-fat hamsters had died by Day 278 of the experiment, possibly of boredom, or maybe shock at the meals the high fat team were getting, or grief at their polyunsaturated colleagues' passing—we don't know.

Unbelievably, it wasn't until Day 361 that the Grim Hamster finally reaped fully half of the hi-life, high saturated fat hamsters. Day 361 instead of day 260 was when deaths in team high-fat finally reached 50%.

Virtually all the omega-6 team were dead by day 300, but on that day more than 80% of the high-fat hamsters were still partying. Let that sink in for a minute: hamsters following the American Heart Association advice to eat more "healthy" omega-6 polyunsaturated fats were virtually all dead by day 300, while those living on a diet full of "bad" saturated animal fats (mainly lard, but also cocoa butter) were nearly all still alive. In fact the last of their number didn't pass until around day 480. I don't know what that is in hamster-years but 480 is more than 300.

Here's the even bigger surprise, these were all hamsters with pre-existing heart failure—the last ones you would recommend a high fat diet to. The ones who nevertheless survived by far the longest were those eating a high saturated fat diet.

You can imagine the shock at Hamster Research HQ. Who was going to break the bad news to the AHA? It could pontificate all it

Oxford Journals, First published online: 29 September 2011 DOI: http://dx.doi.org/10.1093/cvr/cvr258 24-32

liked about the theoretical benefits of a polyunsaturated diet but, when the rubber hit the rodent, the implications were inescapable:

"While we hypothesized that a high PUFA diet enriched with both α-linolenic (flaxseed oil) and linoleic acid (omega-6) would improve mitochondrial oxidative capacity, prevent Ca2+-induced MPTP opening, and prolong survival compared with a standard low-fat diet or a high saturated fat diet, our results were very much to the contrary.

"Surprisingly, consumption of the diet high in long-chain saturated fatty acids prolonged life compared with a standard low-fat diet.

"In contrast to our hypothesis, a high PUFA fat diet enriched with α-linolenic acid and linoleic acid from vegetable sources did not improve survival, cardiac mechanical function, or mitochondrial energetics or resistance to MPTP opening.

"Our findings suggest that high intake of both α-linolenic acid and linoleic acid has a negative effect.

"These results show that a high intake of saturated fat improves survival in heart failure compared with a high PUFA diet or low-fat diet."

They tested the diet your health practitioner wants you on, and those taking it died young. The question you need to ask yourself before following advice to go on a low fat diet or using 'cholesterol lowering' margarines (and even the ones that don't make the claim, frankly), is whether you want to be that hamster?

A big Dutch 2016 observational study on nearly 36,000 people backs up the hamster findings that saturated fats actually protect you from heart disease:[198]

---

198 "The association between dietary saturated fatty acids and ischemic heart disease

"Limiting the intake of dietary SFAs is an important compo-nent of recommendations for the prevention of ischemic heart disease (IHD). High SFA intake is associated with higher blood LDL-cholesterol levels, an established risk factor for IHD.

"*However, the association between SFAs and IHD is now heav-ily debated,* in part because evidence on this link appears to originate mainly from results of early ecologic studies, second-ary prevention studies, and short-term biomarker studies, whereas a direct link between SFAs and IHD in prospective cohort studies is lacking."

That said, they ran the figures and found "total SFA intake was associated with a lower IHD risk (HR [hazard ratio] per 5% of energy: 0.83; 95% CI: 0.74, 0.93)."

What that means is that for every 5% of your energy diet that you filled with saturated fats, you reduced your heart disease risk by 17%. Incredible stuff.

Following official advice and replacing saturated fats with omega-6 PUFAs or carbohydrates, "was significantly associ-ated with higher IHD risks (HR per 5% of energy: 1.27–1.37)."

That's a 27% to 37% increased risk from moving away from animal fats to an omega-6 or high carb diet.

An Australian team of researchers have also looked at the best way to increase omega-3 levels in your blood, and particularly whether you should take your fish oils as part of an omega-6 rich diet, or a saturated fat diet. They noted in the 2016 study that no one else had explored this question yet.[199]

---

depends on the type and source of fatty acid in the European Prospective Investigation into Cancer and Nutrition-Netherlands cohort," Praagman et al, *Am J Clin Nutr* 2016;103:356-65 doi:10.3945/ajcn.115.122671.

199 Saturated Fat Enhances Incorporation Of N-3 Polyunsaturated Fatty Acids Into Plasma

They organised a randomised controlled trial where participants were given a daily fish oil supplement at 2.4g/day. Half
the participants were placed on a high omega-6 diet like the
AHA recommends for six weeks, and the other half were on
a diet high in saturated fats (the kind the health police hate).

Blood analysis at the end of the trial shocked them. People
taking fish oils as part of a high fat diet boosted their omega-3
EPA levels by double, compared to those taking the same fish
oils with omega-6. The DHA increase was also greater for
those on saturated fat.

Conversely, plasma levels of DPA dropped by twice as much
in the omega-6 group. The researchers concluded that a diet of
saturated fat enhanced the bioavailability of omega-3 supplements, whereas a diet of polyunsaturated oils and margarines
did not help. This may also explain the differing results of fish
oil trials—it all depends what you take them with.

Let's make one thing abundantly clear: you do need omega-6
in your diet. It is essential, and there are other benefits from wholegrains that no-one is denying. However, you are consuming so
much omega-6 that it's worth ditching margarine in favour of
butter or an olive oil spread, and ditching polyunsaturated oils
in favour of monounsaturated olive oil, whilst boosting your
omega-3 intake. Ask your local takeaway what oil they use, and
urge olive oil or another monounsaturated variety.

That's the side of the ledger regarding the oversupply of
omega-6 in the diet. The other side regarding omega-3s and
specific benefit is slightly murky. The studies all agree that

And Erythrocyte Lipids In Healthy Humans C.B. Dias et al, Abstracts / *Journal of Nutrition & Intermediary Metabolism* 4 (2016) 6-47

if you take your fish oils via the pan, with a sprig of parsley and a dash of lemon, you get heart protection. Critics of fish oil supplements however, have jumped on three big recent randomised controlled trials that appeared to show no cardio benefit from the purified oil capsules.

The studies, however, were all done on people already with serious heart conditions, so they're known in the industry as 'secondary' trials because they investigate whether the supplements can stave off further problems in people who have already suffered a primary event. A massive primary trial to see whether fish oil pills can prevent heart problems in the first place, the VITAL study, is still ongoing.

In the 17 years since Italy's GISSI trial first found protection against further heart attacks, the medical approach to heart failure has changed with technology and drug improvements. In these three latest trials that poured cold water on the supplements, the heart patients were fully pharmaceuticalised, meaning, as reviewers noted, that any impact of fish oil supplements could have been masked by the drugs. Having said that, in one of the biggest of the trials[200] researchers included a hefty dose of omega-6 with the omega-3s at a ratio of 28:1, meaning there was no way it was going to improve the omega ratio in the patient. In fact it would worsen it. I would have bet money on the outcome before that study even began. Had the research team properly understood that the theory behind omega-3s is balancing out omega-6, they would never have designed their study the way they did. It may have been published in the prestigious *New*

---

200 "n-3 Fatty Acids and Cardiovascular Outcomes in Patients with Dysglycemia," The ORIGIN Trial Investigators* *N Engl J Med* 2012; 367:309-318July 26, 2012DOI: 10.1056/NEJMoa1203859

England Journal of Medicine, but its flaws rendered it as useful as a high school science project. Millions of dollars of research and person hours wasted in my view.

A big meta analysis of 14 random trials noted the flawed study was one of the largest, accounting for 12,500 of the 32,000 total sample, and when this study was left out of their calculations it "led to the statistical reduction of major cardiovascular events."[201] In other words, once the dodgy study was put to one side, the balance of the other studies proved heart benefits from omega-3 supplements:

"[Fish oil supplementation] does exert beneficial effects in reducing death from cardiac causes, sudden cardiac death and death from all causes," the 2014 review of 14 clinical trials concluded.

A cohort study of more than 70,000 Americans over six years taking part in the VITAL diet and lifestyle survey found those taking fish oils or eating fatty fish had reduced risk of 18% for all-cause mortality, 23% reduction in cancer mortality and 13% reduction in cardio deaths.[202]

Even so, not everyone is convinced fish oils are as good as fish. In a cutting assessment of the limitations of fish oil capsules, Paul Clayton of the Institute of Food, Brain & Behaviour in England summarised it thus:[203]

"While the Inuit diet was highly cardio-protective and con-

---

201 "META-ANALYSIS Effects of Omega-3 fatty acid on major cardiovascular events and mortality in patients with coronary heart disease: A meta-analysis of randomized controlled trials," Wen et al, *Nutrition, Metabolism & Cardiovascular Diseases* (2014) 24, 470-475 DOI: http://dx.doi.org/10.1016/j.numecd.2013.12.004
202 "Intake of Long-Chain n-3 Fatty Acids From Diet and Supplements in Relation to Mortality," Bell et al, *Am. J. Epidemiol.* (2014) 179 (6): 710-720. doi: 10.1093/aje/kwt326
203 "From alga to omega; have we reached peak (fish) oil?", Paul R Clayton and Szabolcs Ladi, *J R Soc Med* September 2015 vol. 108 no. 9 351-357 doi: 10.1177/0141076815599673

suming oily fish within a Western diet is to a lesser degree, the case for purified fish oil supplements is less convincing. Purification of fish oil removes lipophilic polyphenols which likely contribute to the health benefits of oily fish; leaving the n3 highly unsaturated fatty acids exposed and prone to conferring oxidative and inflammatory stress. The authors believe that due to such issues as dietary shift, it may now be inadvisable to prescribe or sell purified n 3 highly unsaturated fatty acids supplements, unless the appropriate co-factors are included."

Another major review of more than 200 studies concludes omega-3 supplements from fish and animal sources probably do benefit the heart, and also the brain—in case everyone had forgotten:[204]

"Finally, the cardiovascular system is not the only site of n 3 PUFA action. The brain and retina have the highest levels of DHA of all cell types; ~ 50% of all acyl chains contain DHA. Depletion of the body of n 3 PUFA leads to the replacement of DHA with 22:5, n 6. This minor change in fatty acid structure (22:6, n 3 to 22:5, n 6) in n 3 PUFA deficiency is sufficient to alter visual acuity and cognitive function[205]."

In plain English, if your body is low in omega-3s it plugs the gap with omega-6, making your eyes go funny and your head spin! And that's probably how it all began for the omega-6 hamsters.

---

204 "Omega-3 fatty acid supplementation and cardiovascular disease: Thematic Review Series: New Lipid and Lipoprotein Targets for the Treatment of Cardiometabolic Diseases," Donald B. Jump et al December 2012 *The Journal of Lipid Research*, 53, 2525-2545. doi: 10.1194/jlr.R027904

205 Catalan J., Moriguchi T., Slotnick B., Murthy M., Greiner R. S., Salem N. Jr.. 2002. Cognitive deficits in docosahexaenoic acid-deficient rats. *Behav. Neurosci.* 116: 1022-1031.

7

The Vitamin D Question

OUR YEARS AGO, when my book *Vitamin D: Is This The Miracle Vitamin?* was published, an average of four thousand studies a year were being released on the sunshine vitamin. Now, a search in Google Scholar reveals more than 22,000 studies on "vitamin D" published in the first seven months of 2016 alone. That's an average of 106 a day.

You will perhaps then forgive an 'eye roll' when a Canadian review of studies (meta-analysis) claimed in 2016 after having reviewed 83 studies (an afternoon's worth of output) that it found no evidence of a vitamin D benefit.[206] Now, granted, some of the studies were themselves meta-analyses meaning they covered multiple studies, but it doesn't change the reality that there's more coming down the pipeline every single hour, and all it takes is one study to make a difference.

---

206 "Vitamin D: A Narrative Review Examining the Evidence for Ten Beliefs," G. Michael Allan, *Journal of General Internal Medicine* July 2016, Volume 31, Issue 7, pp 780-791 doi:10. 1007/s11606-016-3645-y

"Wouldn't it be great if there was a single thing that you or I could do to be healthy that was as simple as taking a vitamin, which seems benign, every day? There is an appeal to it. There is a simplicity to it. But for the average person, they don't need it," Canadian lead-author Michael Allan said in a news release.[207] Allan is the director of Evidence Based Medicine at the University of Alberta's Faculty of Medicine & Dentistry.

He looked at ten areas of research, including cancer, but concluded that only in falls and fractures does there seem to be evidence and, at best, even there vitamin D only has a "minor" impact:

"Even areas that we really thought there was good evidence for benefit early on, don't seem to be bearing out," says Allan. "The one that we probably have the most evidence for is fractures. If you were to take a group of people who were at higher risk of breaking a bone--so had about a 15 per cent chance of breaking a bone over the next 10 years--and treated all of them with a reasonable dose of vitamin D for a decade, you'd prevent a fracture in around one in 50 of them over that time."

"Many people would say taking a drug for 10 years to stop one in every 50 fractures is probably not enough to be meaningful. And that's the best vitamin D gets as far as we know now."

But a review by New Zealand government agency Medsafe points out the dangers of "pooling" broad results from different studies, as you may be trying to compare incompatible data:[208]

"Pooling the results of multiple studies may also mask or outweigh any benefit of the different type (e.g. vitamin D2 vs. vitamin D3, etc), dose, dose regimen or route of administration

---

207 http://www.eurekalert.org/pub_releases/2016-06/uoaf-vdm061616.php
208 http://www.medsafe.govt.nz/profs/class/Agendas/agen56-Vitamin%20D.pdf

of vitamin D used. For instance, Bischoff-Ferrari et al (2009a) analysed data from eight trials (totalling 2,426 participants) and found a significant effect on the risk of falls in both ambulatory and institutionalised older individuals, but only at daily vitamin D doses of above 700 IU/day."

New Zealand's state-run Accident Compensation Corporation has paid for vitamin D supplements to be given to every rest home resident in the country because of proven reductions in falls and the consequent savings in medical treatment. In effect it is one of the biggest intervention trials with elderly people anywhere in the world, and it has reduced falls by 38% in elderly care facilities.[209]

Far from preventing one fracture in every 50 over ten years, the vitamin D intervention in NZ has saved thousands over the last seven years. Figures show 28% of people aged over 85 in NZ require medical treatment for falls each year.[210] Eleven percent of the 85+ group will be hospitalised each year from a fall. The average stay in hospital is 15.5 days. Often the falls cause life to be shortened. Reducing that by 38% is not "minor".

So, if the Canadian review is arguably wrong on that, what other areas is vitamin D showing promise in?

Vitamin D has long been linked to reducing risk of colon or bowel cancer. An experiment on mice infected with cells to cause such cancer and given vitamin D supplements each day found a massive impact on tumours:[211]

---

209 http://www.radionz.co.nz/news/national/216495/acc-says-vitamin-d-use-resulting-in-fewer-falls
210 http://www.hqsc.govt.nz/our-programmes/health-quality-evaluation/projects/atlas-of-healthcare-variation/falls/
211 "Increased dietary vitamin D suppresses MAPK signaling, colitis, and colon cancer," Meeker S, *Cancer Res.* 2014 Aug 15;74(16):4398-408. doi: 10.1158/0008-5472.CAN-13-

"At 16 weeks post infection, 11% of mice fed high vitamin D diet had cancer compared with 41% of mice fed maintenance diet."

In other words, mice that didn't take the vitamin D were nearly four times more likely to develop cancer in a controlled trial.

"These findings suggest that increased dietary vitamin D is beneficial in preventing inflammation-associated colon cancer through suppression of inflammatory responses during initiation of neoplasia or early-stage carcinogenesis."

Likewise in hard-to-treat triple negative breast cancer, scientists in lab tests have successfully killed tumours via a vitamin D receptor on the cancer cells.[212] This follows earlier studies confirming that vitamin D kills cancer cells by exploding them—a process known as apoptosis.

Nor is it accurate to claim that there is no clinical trial evidence on vitamin D and cancer. In 2007, the University of Nebraska's Joan Lappe published results from a four year long randomised controlled double blind trial of 1179 women taking either vitamin D and calcium supplements or a placebo.[213]

The results stunned the medical profession. Women on vitamin D supplements reduced their risk of developing cancer in the first 12 months of the study by 77%, compared to women on placebo. Over the whole four years they reduced their cancer risk by 60% compared to the control group.

Researchers have now taken that randomised trial data one

2820. Epub 2014 Jun 17.

212 *Breast Cancer Res Treat.* 2016 May;157(1):77-90. doi: 10.1007/s10549-016-3807-y. Epub 2016 Apr 27. "Vitamin D and androgen receptor-targeted therapy for triple-negative breast cancer." Thakkar et al

213 "Vitamin D and calcium supplementation reduces cancer risk: results of a randomized trial," Lappe et al, *American Journal of Clinical Nutrition* June 2007 vol. 85 no. 6 1586-1591 http://ajcn.nutrition.org/content/85/6/1586.full.pdf+html

step further. They've pooled some of the data from the Lappe study with data from another big study. What they were looking at was the actual blood levels of vitamin D. In Lappe's research the median was 30ng/ml (75 nmol). In a more recent study, the median blood level was 48 ng/ml (120 nmol).

If the vitamin D theory is correct, they theorised, we should expect to see even lower cancer rates in the group whose vitamin D levels were higher. Sure enough, that's exactly what their 2016 study has found. The rate of cancer in Lappe's study after age-adjustment was 1020 cases per 100,000 person-years. In the second study with higher vitamin D that rate dropped to 722/100,000 py's.[214]

Empirical proof, if you still doubt, that vitamin D protects against cancer. After crunching the numbers, scientists found women with vitamin D levels above 40 ng/ml (100 nmol) reduced their risk of cancer by 67% compared to women with blood levels below 20 ng/ml (50 nmol).

"We have quantitated the ability of adequate amounts of vitamin D to prevent all types of invasive cancer combined, which had been terra incognita until publication of this paper," said Cedric Garland, Ph.D, adjunct professor at the University of California (UC) San Diego School of Medicine, Department of Family Medicine and Public Health and member of Moores Cancer Center at UC San Diego Health, and co-author of the study, in a magazine interview.

"These findings support an inverse association between

---

214 McDonnell SL, Baggerly C, French CB, et al. "Serum 25-hydroxyvitamin D concentrations ≥40 ng/ml are associated with >65% lower cancer risk: pooled analysis of randomized trial and prospective cohort study [published online ahead of print April 6, 2016]". *PLoS One.* doi:10.1371/journal.pone.0152441.

25(OH)D and risk of cancer and highlight the importance for cancer prevention of achieving a vitamin D blood serum concentration above 20 ng/mL, the concentration recommended by the IOM for bone health."

Or, as the study itself concluded, high vitamin D levels are "associated with substantial reduction in risk of all invasive cancers combined."

All of which makes the comments of Canada's vitamin D 'Grinch', Professor Mike Allan, look a little dated: "The 40 year old person is highly unlikely to benefit from vitamin D," says Allan. "And when I say highly unlikely, I mean it's not measurable in present science."[215]

If that was true, however, we wouldn't expect to see massive reductions in actual cancer incidences, nor would we expect to keep seeing those magic 60%-70% figures popping up in studies featuring different groups of people.

An Iranian study is a perfect example. A hundred and thirty-five women with breast cancer were matched with 135 healthy women by age and menopause status as a control group.[216]

"Women in the fourth quartile [highest level] of serum vitamin D level were found three times less likely to develop breast cancer, than those in the first quartile," reported *Food Consumer*.

"In an adjusted model, serum vitamin D was inversely associated with the risk for breast cancer, those in the highest levels were 70% less likely to develop the disease, compared to those in the lowest levels.

215 16-Jun-2016 "Vitamin D may not be the great solution to health problems: UAlberta review finds little evidence for the benefits of vitamin D supplementation" news release
216 Jamshidinaeini Y, Akbari ME, Abdollahi M, Ajami M, Davoodi SH. Vitamin D Status and Risk of Breast Cancer in Iranian Women: A Case-Control Study. *J Am Coll Nutr.* 2016 Jun 22:1-8.

"The inverse association was only significant among pre-menopausal women.

"Dietary intake of vitamin D was also inversely associated with risk of breast cancer. Those in the highest quartile were found at nearly 60% reduced risk for breast cancer than those in the lowest quartile. This inverse association was still significant even after adjustment for confounders."

Even on melanoma, the poster-child of the anti-sunshine arm of dermatology, the news is the same. In an article headlined "Vitamin D and Melanoma: What Do We Tell Our Patients?" oncologists discussed the uncomfortable finding that melanoma patients who don't take the sunshine vitamin are much more likely to die from their cancer:[217]

"Patients with melanoma who had a level less than 16 ng/ml were 1.62 times more likely (62% increased risk) to experience recurrence and were 1.76 times more likely to die (76% increased risk) as a result of melanoma.[218] These results closely mirror another recently published, large, cohort study from England, in which patients with 25-hydroxyvitamin D levels (not adjusted for C-reactive protein level) less than 20 nmol/L (8 ng/ml) were 1.52 times more likely than those with higher levels to die as a result of melanoma.[219]"

The irony that staying out of the sun was killing their patients wasn't lost on the doctors, which leads to a brief two minute

---

217 "Vitamin D and Melanoma: What Do We Tell Our Patients?" Sondak et al, *Journal of Clinical Oncology*, VOLUME 34 • NUMBER 15 • MAY 20, 2016, pp 1713-1714

218 Fang S, Sui D, Wang Y, et al: Association of vitamin D levels with outcome in patients with melanoma after adjustment for C-reactive protein. *J Clin Oncol* 34:1741-1747, 2016

219 Newton-Bishop JA, Davies JR, Latheef F, et al: 25-Hydroxyvitamin D2/D3 levels and factors associated with systemic inflammation and melanoma survival in the Leeds melanoma cohort. *Int J Cancer* 136:2890-2899, 2015

diversion: melanoma may not actually be caused by the sun. A growing number of studies are suggesting TV and radio broadcast signals, and mobile phone use, may be causing the radiation damage behind rising rates of melanoma.

Two centuries ago, there were no high frequency radiation transmissions. Today, there are.

"The lifelong incidence of a patient developing skin cancers has been increasing," reports one US study,[220] "and much of the damage done to the skin occurs in a patient's younger years. In 1935, 1 in 1500 children had a lifetime risk of developing melanoma compared with children born today who face a 1 in 33 risk of developing this form of cancer over the course of their life."

Children born today have a risk of melanoma 45 times higher than their grandparents had, yet the sun has not become 45 times more powerful, and for most of the past forty years we have been using sunscreen. In 1935, there were no sunscreens and children played outside because there were no TV or FM radio broadcasts. Today, there are.

Every TV channel signal in your region is ripping through your body before it gets to the TV set. Thousands of mobile calls and data bursts are likewise tearing through the air around you on their way to and from mobile handsets in your region. Miley Cyrus is punching a wrecking ball through your gut every time a classic hits FM station plays it, and not just because you are reacting to the lyrics.

Now it may be that this electromagnetic radiation is not

---

220 Pediatric Sunscreen and Sun Safety Guidelines," Julian et al, Published online before print June 29, 2015, doi: 10.1177/0009922815591889 *CLIN PEDIATR October 2015 vol. 54 no. 12 1133-1140*

doing anything to you. Or it might be that there is so much electronic 'noise' around us that meaningful scientific tests are impossible—who would be an unaffected control group?

Even so, there are still some tests you can do. Transmissions are strongest closest to source, so you would expect to see a cluster effect close to radiation sources.

"A strong association was highlighted between local melanoma incidence and the number of locally covering main Frequency Modulation (FM) transmitters in Sweden," reports one 2016 study before adding, "Twenty-three different European countries were asked to disclose the number of main transmitters used for the FM broadcasting band (87.5-108 MHz) in the respective country. Incidences of melanoma, breast cancer and all cancers together per country were correlated with their respective average density of transmitters."[221]

"Dolk et al.[222] found that there was significant decline in skin and bladder cancer incidence among adults in England as distance from a frequency modulation (FM) broadcasting tower increased."

Then there's this:

"A study performed by doctors from the German city of Naila monitored 1000 residents who had lived in an area around two cell phone towers for 10 years. During the last 5 years of the study they found that those living within 400 meters of either tower had a newly-diagnosed cancer rate three times higher than those who lived further away. Breast cancer

221 "Cancer incidence vs. FM radio transmitter density." Hallberg Ö. *Electromagn Biol Med.* 2016 Jun 29:1-5. [Epub ahead of print] DOI: 10.3109/15368378.2016.1138122
222 Dolk H, Shaddik G, Walls P, et al. Cancer incidence near radio and television transmitters in Great Britain. I and II. *Am J Epidemiol* 1997; 145:1-17

topped the list, but cancers of the prostate, pancreas, bowel, skin melanoma, lung and blood cancer were all increased."[223]

This causation by radio waves may also explain why melanoma usually appears in places on your body where the sun don't shine, and why sunscreens don't offer any proven protection from melanoma.

Hang on, I can hear people saying—sunscreens don't work??

In recent years, reports a 2015 Italian medical study, "many researchers have epidemiologically studied whether sunscreen use influences the malignant melanoma (MM) incidence upon sun exposure. Surprisingly, most of the researchers observed that sunscreen users have a *higher* incidence of MM than non-users."[224]

Add that to the growing list of things the health authorities aren't telling you.

An unbiased 2016 US government NCBI review for health professionals of sunscreen efficacy (which incidentally trashed the credibility of the single sunscreen study from the last 40 years claiming melanoma protection) was equally blunt—just because a sunscreen stops you burning does not mean it is also shielding you from melanoma. It isn't:[225]

"Results from a collaborative European case-control study and one animal study suggest that sunscreens that protect

223 Kaushal, Mohit, Tanvir Singh, and Amit Kumar. "Effects of Mobile Tower Radiations & Case Studies from different Countries Pertaining the Issue." *International Journal of Applied Engineering Research* 7.11 (2012): 1252-1255.
224 "Are tyrosinase inhibitors in sunscreens and cosmetics enhancing UV carcinogenicity?", Morpurgo et al, *Experimental Dermatology*, 2015, 24, 546-559, DOI: 10.1111/exd.12715
225 *Skin Cancer Prevention (PDQ®) Health Professional Version,* PDQ Screening and Prevention Editorial Board.
Published online: April 8, 2016. http://www.ncbi.nlm.nih.gov/books/NBK66059/

against sunburn may not protect against UV radiation–associated cutaneous melanoma...

"A meta-analysis of 18 studies that explored the association between melanoma risk and previous sunscreen use illustrates widely differing study qualities and suggests little or no association.[226] A systematic review of the association between sunscreen use and the development of melanocytic nevi in children reported similar issues with study quality and heterogeneity, hindering conclusive assessments; however, of 15 studies meeting inclusion criteria, 12 found either an increased incidence or no association.[227]

"*Thus, the current evidence indicates that sunscreen application as practiced in the general population shows no clear association with reduced risk of melanocytic nevi or melanoma.*"

Straight from the horse's mouth—or in this case the US National Center for Biotechnology Information. Sounds like some "evidence-based medicine" researchers should take a closer look at sunscreen public health messages. If the stuff doesn't protect from melanoma, why are the public being conned out of $35 a bottle for white snake oil that actually could be killing them by causing a false sense of security? And why were the media jumping all over Australian paleo chef Pete Evans for daring to question the Emperor's new sunscreen lotion?

You may be asking the question, "why would sunscreen users have a higher rate of melanoma?" Well, if vitamin D theory

---

226 Dennis LK, Beane Freeman LE, VanBeek MJ: Sunscreen use and the risk for melanoma: a quantitative review. *Ann Intern Med* 139 (12): 966-78, 2003
227 de Maleissye MF, Beauchet A, Saiag P, et al.: Sunscreen use and melanocytic nevi in children: a systematic review. *Pediatr Dermatol* 30 (1): 51-9, 2013 Jan-Feb.

on cancer is correct, as randomised trials suggest, people who don't use sunscreen have higher vitamin D levels and therefore lower rates of cancer including melanoma. It is also probable, based on the science to date, that people who use sunscreen stay in the sun longer, and if it doesn't actually block the rays that might cause melanoma then it doesn't take a rocket scientist to figure out it's like being on the bridge of the *Starship Enterprise* facing photon torpedoes without realising your shields are down.

Speaking of evidence-based medicine, Professor Allan's Canadian study also came down conclusively against vitamin D for mental health:

"Evidence does not support vitamin D supplementation.... for improving depression/mental well-being."

Yet on the issue of depression, a joint Melbourne University/ Harvard University review in 2016 of 40 clinical trials has found supplements of vitamin D and omega-3 fish oils can "supercharge" the effectiveness of antidepressant medications. Their word, not mine.

"This is an exciting finding because here we have a safe, evidence-based approach that could be considered a mainstream treatment.

"A large proportion of people who have depression do not reach remission after one or two courses of antidepressant medication," Dr Sarris says in a university media release.[228]

"Millions of people in Australia and hundreds of millions worldwide currently take antidepressants. There's real poten-

---

228 "Supplements supercharge antidepressants: Review of 40 clinical trials shows the positive effects of using them in tandem", University of Melbourne, 26 April 2016, https://pursuit.unimelb.edu.au/articles/supplements-supercharge-antidepressants

tial here to improve the mental health of people who have an inadequate response to them."

"Current evidence," concludes the study, "supports adjunctive use of ...omega-3, and vitamin D with antidepressants to reduce depressive symptoms."[229]

Another area that vitamin D is impacting strongly is athletic performance which, by virtue of trickle-down theory, applies to everyone reading this as well. Repeated studies have shown vitamin D working at a cellular level to repair damage from injury or physical stress. It shows up in studies of athletes because differences in cutting edge performance are easy to measure with obvious benefits for test subjects, but the same process takes place in all of us.

A national judoka squad were placed in two groups, one given a single dose of 150,000 IU and one given a placebo. No one knew who was getting what. Blood tests were taken first and then a fitness test using isokinetic dynamometry. Eight days later the blood and fitness tests were repeated, and the results of the randomised double-blind trial revealed the vitamin D group increased their muscle strength by 13% in one week, from one big dose of vitamin D, compared to members of the judoka squad on placebo.[230]

At the top level of any sport athletes would practically kill to get a 13% muscular boost, let alone legally (vitamin D is not and never will be a banned substance).

229 *American Journal of Psychiatry*, Volume 173, Issue 6, June 01, 2016, pp. 575-587 "Adjunctive Nutraceuticals for Depression: A Systematic Review and Meta-Analyses", Sarris et al, http://dx.doi.org/10.1176/appi.ajp.2016.15091228
230 "Acute Effects of Vitamin D3 Supplementation on Muscle Strength in Judoka Athletes: A Randomized Placebo-Controlled, Double-Blind Trial," Wyon et al, *Clinical Journal of Sport Medicine*: July 2016–Volume 26–Issue 4–p 279-284 doi: 10.1097/JSM.0000000000000264

Under the heading "Clinical Relevance", the researchers advised coaches and team doctors:

"Serum 25(OH)D3 levels of indoor athletes should be monitored throughout the year and especially during winter months. Beneficial responses, in muscle strength and serum 25(OH)D3, to 1 dose of vitamin D3 supplementation can be observed within 1 week of ingestion. Muscle strength is linked to serum 25(OH)D levels."

To give you an example of how this might play out, take America's NBA basketball competition. Of 279 professional NBA players given blood tests, 221 or 79.3% had low or deficient vitamin D levels.[231] What kind of difference to their teams might they have made if they'd taken high-dose vitamin D? Thirteen percent stronger equals higher jumps, faster moves.

Researchers tested 103 university athletes in the southern USA across three different collegiate NCAA programmes. They were blood tested and put through a medley of performance challenges:[232]

"Athletes who had lower vitamin D status had reduced performance scores (P<0.01) with odds ratios of 0.85 (15% less ability than high vitamin D athletes) on the Vertical Jump Test, 0.82 (18% less ability) on the Shuttle Run Test, 0.28 (72% less ability) on the Triple Hop for Distance Test, and 0.23 (77% less) on the 1 RM Squat Test. These findings demonstrate that

231 "Vitamin D Deficiency Among Professional Basketball Players," Matthew P. Fishman, *Orthopaedic Journal of Sports Medicine* July 2016 vol. 4 no. 7, doi: 10.1177/2325967116655742
232 "Compromised Vitamin D Status Negatively Affects Muscular Strength and Power of Collegiate Athletes," Hildebrand et al, *International Journal of Sport, Nutrition and Exercise Metabolism*, Acceptance Date: April 11, 2016 DOI: http://dx.doi.org/10.1123/ijsnem.2016-0052

even NCAA athletes living in the southern US are at risk for vitamin D insufficiency and deficiency and that maintaining adequate vitamin D status may be important for these athletes to optimize their muscular strength and power."

Many studies have also found athletes with higher vitamin D levels recover much faster from injury than those who don't: "Vitamin D deficiency is not only associated with an increased susceptibility to stress fractures, muscular injury, and pain but it can also delay recovery post injury," reported one team recently.[233]

Translate that to your own life: what benefit could you get from being stronger, fitter and more energetic, just from a supplement?

Then there's heart health. A big study of acute 1853 chest pain patients followed them for two years after first hospital admission. Blood test results from first admission were checked.

"Two hundred fifty-five patients with known vitamin D concentrations died. In the multivariable analysis, there was a decrease in total mortality above a cut-off level of 40 nmol/L and a decrease in cardiac death above a cut-off level of 70 nmol/L [HRs of 0.66 (95% CI, 0.50–0.88), p = 0.004 and 0.46 (95% CI, 0.22–0.94), p = 0.034, respectively]."[234]

In plain English, people presenting with acute chest pain and vitamin D levels below 16ng/ml (40 nmol/L), were less likely

---

233 "The Emerging Role of Vitamin D in Sports Physical Therapy: A Review," Daniel S. Kahn, *Critical Reviews™ in Physical and Rehabilitation Medicine* DOI: 10.1615/CritRevPhysRehabilMed.2015013808 pages 1-10

234 Naesgaard PA, León de la Fuente RA, Nilsen ST, et al. Suggested Cut-Off Values for Vitamin D as a Risk Marker for Total and Cardiac Death in Patients with Suspected Acute Coronary Syndrome. *Frontiers in Cardiovascular Medicine.* 2016;3:4. doi:10.3389/fcvm.2016.00004

to survive the next two years from death by any cause, whereas those with vitamin D levels above 70 nmol/L (28ng/ml) cut their risk of fatal heart failure by 54%—more than halving it.

It's a fair bet the survivors were very grateful for their higher vitamin D levels, despite the Canadian naysayers who reckon no-one benefits from vitamin D.

Now, one can argue that it wasn't an RCT. The answer is, it didn't need to be. The point of an RCT is to boost the blood levels of a substance in a given population then wait to see what happens. In this case the blood levels were already specifically known, and so were the outcomes. So strong is the link that the research team proposed setting vitamin D levels on admission as a "marker" for probable mortality of the patient.

In heart studies all over the world, they are finding the same things:

"There is increasing evidence that a low vitamin D status may be an important and hitherto neglected factor of cardio-vascular disease. This review is an overview of the current body of literature, and presents evidence of the mechanisms through which vitamin D deficiency affects the cardiovascular system in general and the heart in particular.

"Available data indicate that the majority of congestive heart failure patients have 25-hydroxyvitamin D deficiency. Furthermore, the low serum 25-hydroxyvitamin D level has a higher impact on hypertension, coronary artery disease an on the occurrence of relevant cardiac events.

"A serum 25-hydroxyvitamin D level below 75 nmol/l (30 ng/l) is generally regarded as vitamin D insufficiency in both adults and children, while a level below 50 nmol/l (20 ng/l) is considered deficiency. Levels below 50 nmol/l (20 ng/l) are linked independently to cardiovascular morbidity and mortality."[235]

An Italian study of 18,689 healthy people proved the point. Again, blood tests were taken at the start and participants followed for four years. During that time 412 began to suffer heart failure, mostly those with low vitamin D who were 78% more likely to develop it:[236]

"Individuals with deficient/insufficient levels of serum Vitamin D showed a higher risk of developing HF (HR: 1.78, 95% CI: 1.07-2.97) than those with normal levels... Deficiency of Vitamin D is associated with a significantly higher risk of HF in a general adult population. This association was not explained by an inflammatory marker such as C-Reactive Protein."

Another area of study is on pregnancy. Studies have shown that pregnant women need high vitamin D levels to give their babies optimum brain development. Low vitamin D babies are more likely to develop psychiatric and behavioural problems:

"Vitamin D deficiency during the perinatal period has been hypothesized to increase risk for several psychiatric disorders in humans," reports a 2016 Greek study. "As newborn vitamin D levels are entirely dependent on maternal vitamin D status, vitamin D deficiency in utero may leave the infant vulnerable to cognitive defects and behavioural problems.

"Few human studies have examined these associations with

---

235 Fanari Z, Hammami S, Hammami MB, Hammami S, Abdellatif A. Vitamin D deficiency plays an important role in cardiac disease and affects patient outcome: Still a myth or a fact that needs exploration? *Journal of the Saudi Heart Association.* 2015;27(4):264-271. doi:10.1016/j.jsha.2015.02.003.
236 Abstract P010: Serum Vitamin D and Risk of Heart Failure: Prospective Results From the Moli-sani Study Costanzo et al, *Circulation.* 2016;133:AP010, published online before print March 1, 2016

inconclusive results. We aimed to investigate the associations of maternal 25-hydroxyvitamin D [25(OH) D] levels with offspring neurodevelopment at 4 years of age, using data from a longitudinal, prospective pregnancy cohort, 'Rhea' study in Crete, Greece.[237]

"We included 471 mother-child pairs. Maternal vitamin D status was estimated by measuring plasma concentration of 25(OH) D at the first prenatal visit (13±2.4 weeks). Cognitive function at 4 years was assessed by means of the McCarthy Scales of Children's Abilities (MSCA). Emotional and behavioural development at 4 years was assessed by means of Strengths and Difficulties Questionnaire (SDQ) and Attention Deficit Hyperactivity Disorder (ADHD) Test. Multivariable linear regression analyses were used to estimate the effect of maternal vitamin D status on child neurodevelopment.

"Results: Maternal vitamin D deficiency during early pregnancy was associated with a significant score increase in total SDQ (b-coef: 2.07, 95%CI: 0.25, 3.89) scale and specifically in peer relationship problems (b-coef: 0.58, 95%CI: 0.03, 1.12) and hyperactivity/inattention (b-coef: 1.15, 95%CI: 0.36, 1.94) subscales at 4 years of age. Similarly maternal vitamin D deficiency was associated with five points increase in the total ADHD score (b-coef: 5.36, 95%CI: 0.75, 9.98), and two points increase in the hyperactivity subscale score (b-coef: 2.26, 95%CI: 0.25, 4.26) at 4 years of age. Maternal thyroid function in pregnancy or maternal obesity did not modify the observed associations.

---

237 "Vitamin D deficiency in pregnancy associates with increased emotional and behavioral problems at preschool age: the Rhea pregnancy cohort, Crete, Greece," Daraki et al *Endocrine Abstracts* (2016) 41 EP136
| DOI:10.1530/endoabs.41.EP136

"Conclusion: Vitamin D deficiency in early pregnancy was associated with increased emotional and behavioural problems at preschool age."

On the strength of studies like these and tens of thousands more, England's Public Health agency recommended 2016 that all UK citizens begin taking daily vitamin D supplements. Enough said, really.

The news, however, is not so good on many of those other natural supplements we take every day, as you are about to discover.

8

Natural Supplements: Do They Work?

So HAVING REVIEWED the evidence for major health conditions and the most widely-used nutrient supplements, where does that leave all the other nutriceuticals we pop each day in the hope of remaining eternally youthful, or at the very least earning just another day above ground?

In the game of life, any advantage we can crib together, especially in desperate times, can be the difference between life and death. Sometimes we can lose perspective. Health practitioners might not even blink before offering a $75,000 course of chemotherapy for cancer that, at best, might give you another four months of life. Yet those same oncologists will roll their eyes and look sideways if you suggest a $3,000 course of intravenous vitamin C, and their incorporated society will issue news releases extolling the immorality of "preying" on cancer patients and giving "false hope" with a $39 natural supplement bottle.

It is certainly true that in the later stages of cancer natural supplements are normally useless. But so is expensive chemotherapy, with its added burden of robbing the patient of dignity and quality of life. Yet the big ticket items of cancer and heart disease have earned the pharmaco-medical industrial complex trillions over the years as patients' wallets are systematically vacuumed clean before they are placed in the ground.

This is not to belittle the often sterling efforts of specialists, doctors and nurses in using every tool at their disposal. It's more a commentary on the fact that Big Pharma controls the game with its drugs and treatment regimens, and on the principle that turkeys never vote for an early Christmas nor does Big Pharma realistically want to see a major drop in the number of patients comprising its income stream.

I had a taste of the backlash when I was being interviewed on the radio about vitamin D's proven record of reducing the risk of cancer. The radio station received an email from a purportedly anonymous hotmail account calling vitamin D 'quackery' and urging the station not to promote its use. I was forwarded the email to comment on, and managed to discover the hotmail address had been used on a web forum a year earlier by a named individual. When I Googled the name I discovered he was a senior executive with GlaxoSmithKline, the pharma giant involved in cancer treatment research. The idea of the public cutting their cancer risk by even just 30% was apparently anathema and a threat to the bottom line.

When I later researched some of the cancer charities I found they were all heavily sponsored by Big Pharma. The Melanoma charities, who issue media statements each summer advising people to use more sunscreen, turn out to be sponsored by sunscreen companies and Big Pharma (often the same conglomerates). Given that there's no credible evidence sunscreens protect from melanoma, it's a match made in heaven. Sponsor gets to sell useless product as a perceived public health benefit, then pharmaceutical company sells expensive chemotherapy to treat patients who develop melanoma, then some of those get to go to heaven. As *The Lion King* theme puts it, "the circle of life".

A Harvard economist specialising in public health estimated the 2010 dollar cost of treating newly-diagnosed cancer globally was US$300 billion that year. Cardio-pulmonary disease treatment costs were $400 billion.[238]

More cynical people accuse medical researchers of not taking natural alternatives seriously, but as you may have gathered from this book that isn't fair and nor is it true. Many of our medicines derive from natural substances, and scientists are more than happy to research them.

Sometimes the results are promising, sometimes not. Big studies in the 1990s for example found that giving beta carotene and vitamin A supplements to people at risk of lung disease actually caused them to develop cancer at a 28% increased rate. The trial was stopped two years early because of the tragedy it was causing.[239]

Bearing all that in mind, let's examine a few.

---

238 http://www.bloomberg.com/news/articles/2011-06-20/global-rise-in-cancer-cost-300-billion-in-2010-harvard-economist-says
239 Omenn GS, Goodman GE, Thornquist MD, Balmes J, Cullen MR, Glass A *et al.* Effects of a combination of beta carotene and vitamin A on lung cancer and cardiovascular disease. *N Engl J Med* 1996; 334: 1150-1155

Vitamin C

The Chinese are big fans of natural remedies, so the Shandong Intervention Trial was one to watch. Thousands of people in an area with a high degree of gastric cancer were placed in a randomised trial. One group were given a two week course of antibiotics to kill a bacterial infection thought to cause pre-cancerous gastric lesions. A second group were given garlic for seven years. A third group were given vitamins C, E and selenium, and a fourth were on placebo. The natural remedies were not promising.

"In the Shandong Intervention Trial, 2 weeks of antibiotic treatment for *Helicobacter pylori* reduced the prevalence of pre-cancerous gastric lesions, whereas 7.3 years of oral supplementation with garlic extract and oil (garlic treatment) or vitamin C, vitamin E, and selenium (vitamin treatment) did not."[240]

By the time of the 14.7 year follow-up, more results had come in. The group originally treated with just a two week course of antibiotics nearly 15 years earlier had the lowest rates of gastric cancer—the drugs had lowered their risk by 39% compared with the placebo group.

The group who'd been forced to eat garlic for seven years had nothing to show for it besides bad breath—no reduction in cancers. The same went for the vitamin-selenium mix. No impact.

Except, that is, for mortality. The vitamin mix may not have prevented the cancers, but it appears to have made them more survivable:

"Vitamin treatment was associated with a nearly statistically significant reduction in gastric cancer mortality (fully adjusted

---

240 "Randomized Double-Blind Factorial Trial of Three Treatments To Reduce the Prevalence of Precancerous Gastric Lesions," You et al, JNCI *J Natl Cancer Inst* (19 July 2006) 98 (14): 974-983. doi: 10.1093/jnci/djj264

HR = 0.55 with 95% CI = 0.29 to 1.03, P = .06). Vitamin treatment was associated with a statistically significant reduction in gastric or esophageal cancer mortality (fully adjusted HR = 0.51 with 95% CI = 0.30 to 0.87, P = .014)."[241]

Again, in plain English, the vitamin mix taken daily for seven years cut gastric cancer deaths by 45%, and when you added in esophageal cancers that rose to 49%. Garlic had no impact. The research team said the failure of vitamins to prevent cancer—yet dramatically cut the death rate—raised "the possibility that vitamins lower the rate of mortality after the onset of gastric cancers."

The dosage was 500mg of vitamin C, 200 IU of vitamin E and 75mcg of selenium daily for seven years.

However, as the researchers themselves noted, vitamin C has failed to perform in other randomised controlled trials, and they are uncertain whether it was C, E, selenium or the combination responsible. Additionally, they said, blood serum levels of all these nutrients were low in the region being studied, so the results might not apply to those getting a better diet elsewhere.

The issue of whether vitamin C on its own can fight cancer has never been solved. Like vitamin D, lab experiments have shown vitamin C in a Petri dish can kill tumour cells. Unlike vitamin D, which has a wealth of real world studies showing a protective effect, vitamin C has no such studies.

To understand why, a brief history lesson: humans have never enjoyed the ability to generate our own vitamin C internally.

---

241 "Fifteen-Year Effects of Helicobacter pylori, Garlic, and Vitamin Treatments on Gastric Cancer Incidence and Mortality," Ma et al, JNCI *J Natl Cancer Inst* (2012) doi: 10.1093/jnci/djs003

Other animals do, but we have to get ours from dietary sources. Meat-fat is a great source of vitamin C, but in modern times we don't each much animal fat and our source of choice is fruit.

There's possibly a clue in that. Vitamin D also comes from two sources. Plants give us vitamin D2, which is not very bio-available, while meat, fish and sunlight give us vitamin D3, which is much more easily absorbed. In an earlier chapter we saw how omega-3 oils come from plants like flaxseed, which is near useless in the medical trials, or meat and fish (EPA and DHA) which is highly effective. It turns out the plant form of vitamin C is hard for us to absorb as well.

Study after study of oral supplements of vitamin C has failed to find any clinical use for this nutrient. It just doesn't seem to work as an oral supplement.

However, maybe we've been going about it in the wrong way. That Petri dish experiment began killing cancer at a concentration of 1000 micro-mols/L. To put that in perspective a 300mg vitamin C tablet will peak in your blood at around 75 micro-mols/L, nowhere near enough to do anything. That's because the vast bulk of vitamin C taken orally goes down the toilet unused—not because we don't need it but because we can't absorb more than a fraction of each oral dose.

In 2004 scientists experimented with high dose vitamin C. They found the maximum tolerable oral dose was 3000mg (3g) every four hours. But even that only produced blood serum levels of 220 micro-mols/L—still only a fraction of the 1000 micro-mols/L used in the Petri dish.

When they injected vitamin C intravenously, however, at 1250 mg dosage, they achieved much higher serum levels of 885 micro-mols/L.

They concluded their study with an announcement—ignore previous research and begin testing vitamin C again based on intravenous dosing:[242]

"We recognized that oral or intravenous routes could produce substantially different vitamin C concentrations. We report here that intravenous doses can produce plasma concentrations 30- to 70-fold higher than the maximum tolerated oral doses.

"Only intravenous administration of vitamin C produces high plasma and urine concentrations that might have antitumor activity. Because efficacy of vitamin C treatment cannot be judged from clinical trials that use only oral dosing, the role of vitamin C in cancer treatment should be re-evaluated."

The scientists went looking for case studies where doctors had used intravenous C. They found three:[243]

Case One

In August 1995, doctors discovered a tumour on a 51 year old woman's left kidney. It was 9cm in diameter, extending into the renal vein. A CT scan revealed no metastasis (it had not spread). But by March 1996 a CT scan found clusters of 5mm secondary tumours in the chest which, by November that year, had become "multiple cannonball lesions".

"The patient declined conventional cancer treatment and instead chose to receive high-dose vitamin C administered

---

242 "Vitamin C Pharmacokinetics: Implications for Oral and Intravenous Use," Padayatty et al, *Ann Intern Med.* 2004;140(7):533-537. doi:10.7326/0003-4819-140-7-200404060-00010
243 Pad Padayatty, Sebastian J., et al. "Intravenously administered vitamin C as cancer therapy: three cases." *Canadian Medical Association Journal* 174.7 (2006): 937-942.
http://www.integratedhealthclinic.com/assets/byCancerType/Leukemias-Lymphomas/4-CMAJ%202006-174-937.pdf

intravenously at a dosage of 65 g twice per week starting in October 1996 and continuing for 10 months. She also used other alternative therapies: thymus protein extract, N-acetylcysteine, niacinamide and whole thyroid extract. In June 1997 chest radiography results were normal except for one remaining abnormality in the left lung field, possibly a pulmonary scar."

It was astounding. Instead of radiation or chemotherapy, this woman had beaten metastatic kidney cancer with intravenous vitamin C.

She was, however, a smoker. And in 2001 that habit came back to bite her. She developed lung cancer this time and again chose the vitamin C treatment. Only this time the vitamin C was ineffective against lung cancer. She died November 2002.

Under National Cancer Institute "Best Case" Guidelines, she should not have survived the metastatic kidney cancer.

Case Two

This involved a 49 year old man who went to the doctor with a urination problem and was found to have bladder cancer that had already spread to satellite sites. He too chose intravenous vitamin C, receiving 30g twice a week for three months intensively, and then 30g once every six weeks for the next four years.

"Now, 9 years after diagnosis, the patient is in good health with no symptoms of recurrence or metastasis. The patient used the following supplements: botanical extract, chondroitin sulfate, chromium picolinate, flax oil, glucosamine sulfate, α-lipoic acid, Lactobacillus acidophilus and L. rhamnosus and selenium.

"Complete or partial bladder removal is the standard treatment for stage T2 (muscle invasive) bladder cancer, since the presence of muscle invasion appears to be the best predictor of aggressive behaviour. When treated only locally, as in this case, invasive transitional cell bladder cancer almost invariably develops into clinically apparent local or metastatic disease within a short period."

The bottom line is he lived, without chemotherapy and its side effects.

Case Three

In 1996 a 66 year old woman was diagnosed with stage 3 lymphoma, which is normally terminal. After a short radiotherapy treatment she declined chemo in favour of intravenous vitamin C.

"The patient remains in normal health 10 years after the diagnosis of diffuse large B-cell lymphoma, never having received chemotherapy. The patient used additional products: β-carotene, bioflavonoids, chondroitin sulfate, coenzyme Q10, dehydroepiandrosterone, a multiple vitamin supplement, N-acetylcysteine, a botanical supplement and bismuth tablets. Histopathologic examination of the original paraspinal mass at the NIH confirmed a diffuse large B-cell lymphoma at stage III, with a brisk mitotic rate.

"Patients with untreated stage III diffuse B-cell lymphoma have a dismal prognosis. This case, like the preceding one, is unusual in that the patient refused chemotherapy, which might have produced a long-term remission. It appears, nonetheless, that a cure occurred in connection with intravenous vitamin C infusions."

The researchers, from the National Institutes of Health at Bethesda, were at pains to point out that three swallows do not a summer make—it doesn't prove beyond doubt that intravenous C worked, but it is plausible.

It was enough to spark renewed interest in medical circles. A New Zealand review of intravenous C notes that it is pointless trying to take a big dose of vitamin C orally—anything more than 400mg will flush out:[244]

"Saturation of bioavailability mechanisms occurs at oral doses of 400 mg daily equating to blood levels of 60–100µM. IV dosing bypasses this tight control, achieving plasma concentrations up to 20 mM."

In fact clinical trials on cancer patients have dosed them intravenously at rates of 1.5g vitamin C per kilo of bodyweight, achieving blood levels of 26mM (26 millimols or 26000 micromols).[245]

They think the way it works is that intravenous C bypasses the digestive system, allowing high levels of serum in the blood for about four hours before it is processed by the kidneys and eliminated in the body's attempt to balance levels again. During that four hour window, the extremely high levels of ascorbic acid (vitamin C) create hydrogen peroxide in organs and tissues, and it is the hydrogen peroxide that is toxic in that particular circumstance to cancer cells but not ordinary cells.

Taking oral vitamin C is like landing on the go directly to jail space in monopoly, you don't get to collect the cancer-fighting bonus. It's the intravenous dosing that slips it into your system, not oral dosing.

That said, don't believe websites that assure you megadosing on vitamin C is always safe. The New Zealand review found

---

244 "Review of high-dose intravenous vitamin C as an anticancer agent," Wilson et al, *Asia-Pacific Journal of Clinical Oncology* 2014; 10:22-37 doi: 10.1111/ajco.12173
245 Hoffer LJ, Levine M, Assouline S et al. Phase I clinical trial of i.v. ascorbic acid in advanced malignancy. *Ann Oncol* 2008; 19 (11): 1969-1974.

studies where it caused kidney stones, kidney failure, and cases where tumours even seemed to feed on the vitamin C:

"In patients with widespread and rapidly proliferating tumours, vitamin C has been reported to cause tumour acceleration and precipitate tumour haemorrhage and necrosis.[246] [247] The initial Cameron and Campbell trial described four patients in this category.

"Potentially, this could also be explained by the natural history of the underlying cancer. Dyspepsia, nausea and altered bowel habit are the most frequently reported side effects, particularly following oral administration.

"High doses of oral vitamin C have been shown to affect iron absorption and interfere with many routine laboratory parameters. In patients with congestive heart failure and ascites, the high fluid intake associated with administration may exacerbate their condition."

The New Zealand review was comprehensive and lays out a path forward for trialling intravenous C, so it isn't fair to say that medics have not been paying attention. What they do say is that without proper clinical trials, it is too early to recommend it as a stand-alone alternative to chemotherapy. If you want to try IVC, you will need to find a doctor willing to argue your case.

The clinical trials that have taken place combined vitamin C with chemotherapy, and delivered no benefits, but no one has been brave enough to trial IVC on its own.

---

246 Cameron E, Campbell A. The orthomolecular treatment of cancer. II. Clinical trial of high-dose ascorbic acid supplements in advanced human cancer. *Chem Biol Interact* 1974; 9(4): 285-315
247 Campbell A, Jack T. Acute reactions to mega ascorbic acid therapy in malignant disease. *Scott Med J* 1979; 24(2): 151-3.

What are the alternatives?

The only other way of possibly getting high dose vitamin C is a nanotechnology product called "liposomal Vitamin C". It's an oral dose that encapsulates ascorbic acid in liposome particles for claimed better absorption by the body. The manufacturers claim a bioavailability close to intravenous delivery, which obviously opens up the opportunity for DIY cancer treatment.

Unfortunately, a search of Google Scholar reveals a 2016 clinical trial on liposomal vitamin C which is less than impressive. That may seem unfair, because the study was only looking at vitamin C's antioxidant abilities and to that extent the liposomal C did its job. However, when you look at the numbers needed in terms of fighting cancer you'll see what I mean.

The clinical trial tested how a 4g dose of vitamin C affected blood plasma antioxidant levels depending on how it was delivered. One group were given a standard oral dose. Another were given 4g intravenously, while another group were given an oral dose of liposomal C.

All doses, including the standard oral, hit the target level of antioxidant in the blood. However the liposomal dose was only marginally more effective than the oral tablet. Intravenous C on the other hand delivered a truckload more bioavailability:[248]

Intravenous C caused a blood level of "57.0 ± 6.9 (mg/dL" (5038 micromols/L) whereas liposomal vitamin C delivery caused a blood level of "10.3 ± 0.9", (884 micromols/L) and oral C caused blood levels of "7.6 ± 0.4" (672 micromols/L).[249]

---

248 Davis JL, Paris HL, Beals JW, et al. Liposomal-encapsulated Ascorbic Acid: Influence on Vitamin C Bioavailability and Capacity to Protect Against Ischemia-Reperfusion Injury. *Nutrition and Metabolic Insights.* 2016;9:25-30. doi:10.4137/NMI.S39764.
249 "Ascorbic Acid Supplementation: Influence of Delivery Method on Vitamin C

The point of the story? Liposomal vitamin C is better than ordinary C, but it is nowhere near as effective as intravenous C on the most recent clinical trial data. And according to the 2016 trial report, there's only been one other human trial:

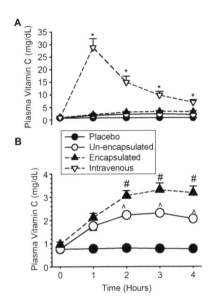

"To our knowledge, there has been only one other published human study evaluating oral delivery of vitamin C encapsulated in liposomes, and this was a pilot study with only two research participants.[250]

"Circulating concentrations of vitamin C following oral delivery of 5 g of vitamin C encapsulated in liposomes were compared with concentrations following 5 g of unencapsulated vitamin C. No discernible differences were detected between the plasma concentrations; however, in light of its status as a pilot study, and with only two research participants, this lack of difference could be attributed to insufficient statistical power, that is, a type 2 error.

"While human studies of liposomal vitamin C may be lacking, the concept and utilization of liposomes for pharmaceutical delivery are well established."

Bioavailability and Capacity to Protect Against Ischemia-Reperfusion Injury," Davis et al, April 2015, *The FASEB Journal* vol. 29 no. 1 Supplement 635.2

250 Hickey S, Roberts HJ, Miller NJ. Pharmacokinetics of oral vitamin C. *J Nutr Environ Med.* 2008;17(3):169-177.

So there it is—despite the hype from some quarters there's no hard clinical evidence yet that megadose vitamin C will kill cancer, although there is evidence that it *could*. Liposomal vitamin C is marginally more bioavailable than ordinary vitamin C tablets, and seems to be the best oral delivery system for vitamin C as an antioxidant. However liposomal C is five times weaker than intravenous vitamin C based on human trials to date.

Another group of researchers argue a paleo approach, pointing out that humans have obtained more vitamin C from meat throughout history than fruit. A hundred grams of cooked pork liver, for example, contains more than double the vitamin C of 100g of cooked spinach.

They, too, reviewed the dismal history of clinical trials of vitamin C: "none of the studies reported a clinically meaningful benefit as regards mortality, incidence of common cold, cardiovascular events, and prevention or treatment of cancer."[251]

Echoing a theory you've already heard in this book, the researchers believe the reason trials for cancer haven't worked is because of other factors. While numerous studies show good blood levels of vitamin C are protective, supplementation always fails to deliver results. Why? Western diets, particularly the long-favoured high carb low fat diet, boost blood sugar. Glucose does two things: it interferes with vitamin C absorption, and it is like pouring petrol on a fire for cancer.

"Cancer cells are highly dependent on glucose and are unable to use fat or ketones for energy, a metabolic failure ketogenic diets are aimed to exploit. We suggest that an animal based, low

---

251 *Journal of Evolution and Health*, Vol. 1 [2013], Iss. 1, Art. 13 http://jevohealth.com/journal/vol1/iss1/13 DOI: 10.15310/2334-3591.1030

carbohydrate high fat diet (instead of the currently used ketogenic diets) may provide vitamin C not only in sufficient amounts but also in a bioavailable form, and thus may be more appropriate for the treatment of cancer as compared with the versions of the classical ketogenic diets that are currently used in clinical trials."

The current dietary guidelines, they point out, rely on fruit for vitamin C intake, "thereby also increasing carbohydrate load and intake of polyphenols which both inhibit vitamin C utilization.

"By contrast, studies of contemporary hunter-gatherer societies as well as documentations of the arctic people from the 18th and 19th century indicate no signs of scurvy despite subsisting on diets predominated by foods of animal origin and using no vitamin supplements. Our own clinical experience with the paleolithic ketogenic diet also shows improving health parameters and long-term sustainability of meat-fat based diet in the absence of vitamin C supplementation.

"Even though the amount of dietary vitamin C consumed on an animal meat-fat based diet may be lower as compared to dietary intake from some fruits and vegetables, the former may ensure a higher bioavailability of vitamin C.

"A mismatch between our current diet and ancestral physiology may explain why deficient levels of vitamin C are associated with disease.

"Instead of supplementing vitamin C, changing our nutrition as a whole and adopting a meat-fat based diet, even if it may sound a radical solution, may be a better choice to support vitamin C homeostasis."

Probably not what you expected to discover, but consistent with the emerging evidence that the so-called "healthy diets" of the past forty years have been killing us.

Take home points:

Taking more than 500mg of ordinary vitamin C a day orally for anything is probably a waste of money.

Intravenous vitamin C could possibly be used in place of chemotherapy (at your own risk), but doesn't appear to work in conjunction with it.

If you have cancer, lower your carb and sugar intake radically.

Avemar

If there is a rising star of natural cancer treatment, it would have to be Avemar, the trade name of a fermented wheat germ extract invented by Hungarian scientist Máté Hidvégi in the 1990s, Avemar is another case of science stumbling across nature and striking gold.

Although it is based on wheat germ cast aside during the bread manufacturing process, simply including wheat germ in your diet won't deliver the benefits. It is the fermentation of the wheat germ with a specific yeast that creates the active chemicals, 2,6-Dimethoxy-p-benzoquinone and 2-methoxybenzoquinone. Which is why they called it Avemar—it is easier to say.

What quickly became apparent is that Avemar kills cancer cells. Not only that, it does so without any side effects.

"Avemar, the product of industrial fermentation of wheat germ, possesses unique cancer-fighting characteristics. Taken orally, Avemar can inhibit metastatic tumour dissemination and proliferation during and after chemotherapy, surgery, or radiation," reports the New York Academy of Sciences.[252]

---

252 "Fermented Wheat Germ Extract (Avemar) in the Treatment of Cancer and Autoimmune Diseases," Boros et al, New York Academy of Sciences, *Ann. N.Y. Acad. Sci.* 1051: 529-542 (2005). doi: 10.1196/annals.1361.097

Hundreds of laboratory tests have taken place using animals and human cancer cell cultures in Petri dishes. No animals have been harmed by Avemar, no humans taking it have been harmed, but breast cancer cells were obliterated.

Scientists treated breast cancer cells with the well known drug tamoxifen, but it wasn't till they added Avemar to the dish that cancer cells began dying left, right and centre in a process known as apoptosis.

"After an exposure time of 48 h, Avemar increased apoptosis significantly...The increase in apoptosis by the combined use of tamoxifen + Avemar suggests that the addition of Avemar to tamoxifen may enhance the efficacy of tamoxifen in ER+ breast cancer. There is no contraindication to their combination in clinical practice."

In a randomised clinical trial in America, melanoma patients given Avemar with their chemotherapy were much more likely (86%) to be cancer free after a seven year follow up than those on chemotherapy alone, and 50% more likely to be alive.[253]

"The inclusion of Avemar into the adjuvant protocols of high-risk skin melanoma patients is *highly* recommended," reported the study authors.

Similar results were reported in a colorectal cancer trial involving 170 patients, one group receiving just chemo, and the other chemo plus Avemar.[254]

---

253 "Adjuvant fermented wheat germ extract (Avemar) nutraceutical improves survival of high-risk skin melanoma patients: a randomized, pilot, phase II clinical study with a 7-year follow-up," Demidov et al, *Cancer Biother Radiopharm.* 2008 Aug;23(4):477-82. doi: 10.1089/cbr.2008.0486.
254 Jakab F, Shoenfeld Y, Balogh A, Nichelatti M, Hoffmann A, Kahan Z et al. A medical nutriment has supportive value in the treatment of colorectal cancer. *Br J Cancer.* 2003;89:465-69 DOI: 10.1038/sj.bjc.6601153

"End-point analysis revealed that progression-related events were significantly less frequent in the MSC [Avemar] group (new recurrences: 3.0 vs. 17.3%, P<0.01; new metastases: 7.6 vs. 23.1%, P<0.01; deaths: 12.1 vs. 31.7%, P<0.01)."

Expressed another way, those *not* given Avemar were almost six times more likely to suffer a recurrence, three times more likely to be told their cancer had spread and two and a half times more likely to die.

"Continuous supplementation of anticancer therapies with MSC for more than 6 months is beneficial to patients with colorectal cancer in terms of overall and progression-free survival."

In another human trial involving 45 patients with Stage 2 and 3 head and neck cancers, those not given Avemar were 12 times more likely to suffer a relapse within a year, (12 patients compared to only one relapse on Avemar), four times more likely to suffer metastasis (four to one), and eight times more likely to be told their cancer had progressed (17 cases to 2).[255]

At the end of five years, 74% of the original Avemar group were still alive. Only 45% of the chemotherapy group were alive. Overwhelmingly, by similar margins across all these trials, Avemar is saving lives.

Additional to its actual anticancer strengths, Avemar also reduces the side effects of chemotherapy, combating nausea and appetite loss.

Reviewing the evidence in 2011, medical scientists stated:[256]

---

255 *Hungarian Medical Journal* 2006 Volume 147, Issue 35, 1709-1711, "The opinion of Hungarian Association of Oral and Maxillofacial Surgeons (Magyar Arc-, Állcsont- és Szájsebészeti Társaság) on the justification of supportive treatment of patients with tumorous diseases of the oral cavity"
256 Fermented wheat germ extract–nutritional supplement or anticancer drug?" Thomas Mueller and Wieland Voigt, *Nutr J.* 2011 Sep 5;10:89

"In conclusion, available data so far justify the use of FWGE as a non-prescription medical nutriment for cancer patients. Further randomized, controlled and large scale clinical studies are mandatory, to further clarify the value of FWGE as a drug component of future chemotherapy regimens."

If you have cancer, reach for Avemar immediately.

Resveratrol

We've all heard about resveratrol by now. One of the active ingredients in red wine, it has long been a suspected agent of influence in the Mediterranean diet paradox. In a 200ml glass of red, expect to find 7mg of resveratrol. On the face of it, that doesn't appear to be a useful dose.

A review of six studies that looked at resveratrol's impact on blood pressure only found doses of higher than 150mg were effective, and only on systolic pressure:

"The overall outcome of the meta-analysis indicates that resveratrol consumption cannot significantly reduce Systolic BP and Diastolic BP. Subgroup analyses indicated that higher-dose of resveratrol consumption ($\geq$150 mg/d) significantly reduces SBP of -11.90 mmHg (95% CI: -20.99, -2.81 mmHg, P = 0.01), whereas lower dose of resveratrol did not show a significant lowering effect on SBP."[257]

The revelation that high doses are needed is because—like nearly all plant-based nutrients we've covered in this book—resveratrol has a poor uptake in the human body leaving you with little bang for your buck:

---

257 Liu, Yanxia, et al. "Effect of resveratrol on blood pressure: a meta-analysis of randomized controlled trials." *Clinical Nutrition* 34.1 (2015): 27-34. doi:10.1016/j.clnu.2014.03.009

"Bioavailability of resveratrol is one of the focal points because the compound is poorly bioavailable, low water soluble, and chemically unstable. After oral administration or intravenous injection of resveratrol in humans, resveratrol was rapidly metabolized within 2 hours, even a peak in 30 minutes. Several studies in vivo in animals and humans demonstrated a very low intestinal uptake of resveratrol, and it was difficult to detect unmetabolized resveratrol in the circulating plasma."[258]

With a half-life of between 8-14 minutes, the resveratrol you take may well have disintegrated into sulfate and other chemicals before it even starts to get pumped by the heart. The "peak" in the blood after half an hour is felt by users as an energy boost and regarded by some researchers as more of a dead cat bounce.

"Trans-resveratrol is photosensitive, is easily oxidized, and presents unfavourable pharmacokinetics. Therefore, successful clinical application of resveratrol is a severe challenge for the medical as well as pharmaceutical technology."[259]

Little surprise, then, that a recent study of 783 village-living Italians found *dietary* resveratrol from grapes, wine, blueberries, peanuts and chocolate had no impact on their health:[260]

"In older community-dwelling adults, total urinary resveratrol metabolite concentration was not associated with inflammatory markers, cardiovascular disease, or cancer or

---

258 Teng Ma, Meng-Shan Tan, Jin-Tai Yu, and Lan Tan, "Resveratrol as a Therapeutic Agent for Alzheimer's Disease," *BioMed Research International*, vol. 2014, Article ID 350516, 13 pages, 2014. doi:10.1155/2014/350516
259 ibid
260 Semba RD, Ferrucci L, Bartali B, et al. Resveratrol Levels and All-Cause Mortality in Older Community-Dwelling Adults. *JAMA Intern Med.* 2014;174(7):1077-1084. doi:10.1001/jamainternmed.2014.1582.

predictive of all-cause mortality. Resveratrol levels achieved with a Western diet did not have a substantial influence on health status and mortality risk of the population in this study."

A well known clinical trial of 500mg resveratrol doses on healthy young people found it improved blood flow to the brain, but had no impact on their mental ability.[261] Nothing like giving teenagers a rush of blood to the head!

So there's a hint of potency about resveratrol. Reading the "pre-clinical" studies done in Petri dishes and animal experiments, it's easy to see why science is excited. Resveratrol performs—in the lab. In real life, however, meaningful evidence is more difficult to come by.

For example, hard on the heels of the blood pressure findings, another review of studies found resveratrol does not lower cholesterol either, although given what's been revealed in this book that may now be irrelevant:[262]

"Overall, resveratrol supplementation had no significant effect on any of the lipid parameters assessed: total cholesterol... low-density lipoprotein cholesterol... high-density lipoprotein cholesterol, and triglycerides. These results were robust in sensitivity analysis and were not dependent on the resveratrol dose, the duration of supplementation, or the cardiovascular risk status of the population studied."

---

261 D. O. Kennedy, E. L. Wightman, J. L. Reay et al., "Effects of resveratrol on cerebral blood flow variables and cognitive performance in humans: a double-blind, placebo-controlled, crossover investigation," *The American Journal of Clinical Nutrition*, vol. 91, no. 6, pp. 1590-1597, 2010

262 Sahebkar, Amirhossein. "Effects of resveratrol supplementation on plasma lipids: a systematic review and meta-analysis of randomized controlled trials." *Nutrition Reviews* 71.12 (2013): 822-835. DOI: http://dx.doi.org/10.1111/nure.12081 822-835 First published online: 1 December 2013

If resveratrol is good for the heart, said the reviewers, it must be happening in some other way.

Another team in 2015 also came up with no cardiovascular benefits:[263]

"This meta-analysis of available RCTs does not suggest any benefit of resveratrol supplementation on CV risk factors."

A recurring theme in this book has been the foolishness of looking at individual food ingredients in isolation. That may be a factor in this case as well. Another study found resveratrol became active at much lower doses when mixed with other red wine polyphenols (RWPs):

"Resveratrol had pro-oxidant or antioxidant effects depending on (lower or higher) dosage. RWP protection from photolipoperoxidation was dose-dependent and increased with dosage. Combination of the two compounds exhibited synergistic antioxidant effect, and made resveratrol effective both at lower and higher dosages.[264]

"These results suggest that resveratrol requires red wine polyphenols for optimum antioxidant activity."

One area where resveratrol has definitely come into its own is bone disease. A randomised controlled trial involving 74 men at risk of losing bone mass dosed up to 1g/day vs. placebo. CT scans revealed a significant increase in bone mass among the resveratrol group.[265]

---

263 Sahebkar, Amirhossein, et al. "Lack of efficacy of resveratrol on C-reactive protein and selected cardiovascular risk factors–Results from a systematic review and meta-analysis of randomized controlled trials." *International journal of cardiology* 189 (2015): 47-55. doi:10.1016/j.ijcard.2015.04.008

264 "Resveratrol requires red wine polyphenols for optimum antioxidant activity," Cavallini, G., Straniero, S., Donati, A. et al. *J Nutr Health Aging* (2016) 20: 540. doi:10.1007/s12603-015-0611-z

265 "Resveratrol Increases Bone Mineral Density and Bone Alkaline Phosphatase in Obese

"Our data suggest that high-dose RSV supplementation positively affects bone, primarily by stimulating formation or mineralization. Future studies of longer duration comprising populations at risk of osteoporosis are needed to confirm these results."

Such findings also have relevance to victims of bone cancers like multiple myeloma. Lab studies had shown resveratrol killed myeloma cells *in vitro*. That finding led to human trials on people with multiple myeloma. It was an unmitigated disaster.

Knowing that normal dietary supplements were incapable of delivering resveratrol into the bloodstream fast enough, the trial used a modified form (SRT501) developed by Sirtris Pharmaceutical Laboratories to deliver higher bioavailability.[266]

"15 of 24 patients treated with SRT501 monotherapy [micronized resveratrol on its own]were withdrawn from treatment (10 due to AEs [adverse events], 1 due to AE leading to death and 4 following investigator's decision). All nine patients receiving SRT501 and bortezomib [resveratrol and chemo combined] were withdrawn from study (5 due to AEs, 3 following investigator's decision and one patient withdrawal).

"The predominant study finding was unexpected renal toxicity, with five SAEs [serious adverse events] of renal failure leading to early study termination.

"All five patients reported nausea and vomiting prior to hospitalization and two required temporary haemodialysis. Renal biopsy performed in two patients demonstrated cast and

Men: A Randomized Placebo-Controlled Trial", Ornstrup et al, *Clin Endocrinol Metab,* December 2014, 99(12):4720-4729, doi: 10.1210/jc.2014-2799

266 Popat, R., Plesner, T., Davies, F., Cook, G., Cook, M., Elliott, P., Jacobson, E., Gumbleton, T., Oakervee, H. and Cavenagh, J. (2013), A phase 2 study of SRT501 (resveratrol) with bortezomib for patients with relapsed and or refractory multiple myeloma. *British Journal of Haematology,* 160: 714-717. doi: 10.1111/bjh.12154

crystal nephropathy in one, and acute tubular damage without cast nephropathy in the other. Disease progression occurred in four of the five patients at the time of renal failure and two patients were discharged for palliation [hospice care]. Following three cases, a medical review meeting recommended further monitoring and recruitment was stopped following five SAEs."

In the shakedown that followed, scientists noted that a previous SRT501 trial on colorectal cancer patients had not caused kidney failure—but multiple myeloma patients appeared particularly vulnerable to this side effect. This was a major blow given resveratrol's test-tube success at killing myeloma tumours and proven trial success at rebuilding bone density. Further proof, if needed, that real life clinical trials are far more complex than merely isolating one ingredient.

Researchers followed that up with more bad news, this time a resveratrol trial on mice with multiple sclerosis, a disease that strips protective coverings off nerves. Far from helping, resveratrol made it worse:[267]

"Surprisingly, the resveratrol treatment significantly exacerbated demyelination and inflammation without neuroprotection in the central nervous system in both models. Our findings indicate that caution should be exercised in potential therapeutic applications of resveratrol in human inflammatory demyelinating diseases, including multiple sclerosis."

Other small clinical trials on healthy people have found resveratrol generally well-tolerated, and capable of influencing cancer cells, but paradoxically also capable of interfering

---

267 Sato, Fumitaka, et al. "Resveratrol exacerbates both autoimmune and viral models of multiple sclerosis." *The America Journal of Pathology* 183.5 (2013): 1390-1396. doi:10.1016/j.ajpath.2013.07.006

with medication. The size of the studies raises doubts about their statistical power to determine much beyond coincidence, however. Commenting on that, and the myeloma tragedy, one review concluded:[268]

"From this limited clinical trial data, it is apparent that much more human research is needed before resveratrol can be considered as a viable option for cancer prevention or therapy."

The review then went through the many conflicting experiments on animals before lamenting:

"There is little evidence from animal or human studies that resveratrol can serve as a viable treatment option once tumours are already formed, so it is not likely that resveratrol can be used as an alternative for the traditional forms of cancer treatment in the near future.... However, there is some promising evidence that resveratrol can improve metabolic outcomes and could have a major impact on overall health, including decreasing cancer risk."

Provided they get the dose right, presumably, and figure out how to get it inside the body efficiently.

As a 2016 review warned, "The notion of resveratrol as a "magic bullet" was recently challenged by clinical trials showing that this polyphenol does not have a substantial influence on health status and mortality risk."[269]

A 2014 review, spanning nearly 40 pages, was entitled: "Resveratrol and cardiovascular health—Promising therapeutic

268 "Resveratrol and cancer: focus on in vivo evidence," Carter et al, doi: 10.1530/ERC-13-0171 *Endocr Relat Cancer June 1, 2014 21 R209-R225*
269 "Resveratrol: How Much Wine Do You Have to Drink to Stay Healthy?", Sabine Weiskirchen and Ralf Weiskirchen doi: 10.3945/an.115.011627 *Adv Nutr July 2016 Adv Nutr vol. 7: 706-718, 2016*

or hopeless illusion?" The authors, calling it an investigation into resveratrol's "putative" benefits, decided not to embroil themselves further in the fight:[270]

"Because the body of work encompassing the stilbenes and other phytochemicals in the context of longevity and the ability to presumably mitigate a plethora of afflictions is replete with conflicting information and controversy, especially so with respect to the human response, we tried to remain as neutral as possible in compiling and presenting the more current data with minimal commentary, permitting the reader free reign to extract the knowledge most helpful to their own investigations."

Hugely frustratingly for researchers, studies on red wine itself continue to show health benefits, raising the question yet again about taking single ingredients out of context. More than 5000 Norwegians were studied for seven years:

"Moderate wine consumption was independently associated with better performance on all cognitive tests in both men and women. There was no consistent association between consumption of beer and spirits and cognitive test results. Alcohol abstention was associated with lower cognitive performance in women.

"Conclusions – Light-to-moderate wine consumption was associated with better performance on cognitive tests after 7 years follow up."[271]

---

270 "Resveratrol and cardiovascular health–Promising therapeutic or hopeless illusion?" Tang et al, *Pharmacological Research* Volume 90, December 2014, Pages 88-115, doi:10.1016/j.phrs.2014.08.001

271 Arntzen KA, Schirmer H, Wilsgaard T, Mathiesen EB. Moderate wine consumption is associated with better cognitive test results: a 7 year follow up of 5033 subjects in the Tromsø Study. *Acta Neurol Scand:* 2010: 122 (Suppl. 190): 23-29. DOI: 10.1111/j.1600-0404.2010.01371.x

The emphasis is on "light". A study of nearly 20,000 Danish alcoholics reveals heavy drinking nearly triples your risk of heart disease or stroke.[272] If you've got resveratrol in the cupboard, the evidence shows it is still worth taking as an antioxidant, and particularly in combination with other ingredients like astaxanthin, green tea or co-enzyme Q10. Medical science has not given up on resveratrol, they're just trying to figure out how to turn lab success into reality inside actual human beings.

Selenium

Another essential element, but only in moderation. Commonly found in meat, fish, mushrooms and nuts. Some countries, like New Zealand, have low levels of selenium in the soil so nutritionists sometimes recommend Brazil nuts or supplements. The only problem is that high selenium levels in men have now been linked to a 91% increase in the risk of prostate cancer—already one of the leading fatal cancers in men.[273] The advice from urologists to men is blunt: "Evidence suggests supplements with vitamin E and/or selenium should be avoided".[274]

The men in the study had strong serum levels of selenium (median 172 ng/ml) before starting that trial, so the supple-

---

272 "Incidence of cardiovascular and cerebrovascular disease in Danish men and women with a prolonged heavy alcohol intake," Hvidtfeldt et al, *Alcohol Clin Exp Res.* 2008 Nov;32(11):1920-4. doi: 10.1111/j.1530-0277.2008.00776.x. Epub 2008 Aug 18.
273 Kristal AR, Darke AK, Morris JS, et al. Baseline selenium status and effects of selenium and vitamin E supplementation on prostate cancer risk. *J Natl Cancer Inst* 2014;106:djt456
274 Marra, Giancarlo, Marco Oderda, and Paolo Gontero. "Dietary supplements and prostate cancer prevention." *Trends in Urology & Men's Health* 7.1 (2016): 12-16. http://onlinelibrary.wiley.com/doi/10.1002/tre.500/pdf

ment was boosting levels even higher. There is evidence of a sweet spot for selenium however, with another randomised trial of 200 micrograms a day showing it halved the development of non-aggressive prostate cancer in men with low selenium levels going in:

"Selenium Supplementation (SS) continued to significantly reduce the overall incidence (relative risk and 95% confidence interval) of prostate cancer (0.51, 0.29–0.87). The protective effect of SS appeared to be confined to those with a baseline PSA level of ≤ 4 ng/mL (0.35, 0.13–0.87), although the inter-action of baseline PSA and treatment was not statistically significant. Participants with baseline plasma selenium con-centrations only in the lowest two tertiles (< 123.2 ng/mL) had significant reductions in prostate cancer incidence. A significant interaction between baseline plasma selenium and treatment was detected."[275]

Those studies above were looking at whether selenium could prevent cancer. But a big 2015 review looked at whether sele-nium as a natural supplement could help treat men with pros-tate cancer *after* diagnosis. The answer is an emphatic 'no!'; if you have prostate cancer and start taking selenium, you can nearly triple your chance of dying. It showed up on a sliding scale: those who supplemented above ordinary diet by 24 micrograms a day increased their risk by 18%, a dose between 25mcg and 140mcg boosted fatality rates by 33%, and taking

---

275 Duffield-Lillico, A.J., Dalkin, B.L., Reid, M.E., Turnbull, B.W., Slate, E.H., Jacobs, E.T., Marshall, J.R., Clark, L.C. and for the Nutritional Prevention of Cancer Study Group (2003), Selenium supplementation, baseline plasma selenium status and incidence of prostate cancer: an analysis of the complete treatment period of the Nutritional Prevention of Cancer Trial. *BJU International*, 91: 608-612. doi: 10.1046/j.1464-410X.2003.04167.x

more than 140mcg/day put men 2.6 times more likely to die than men not taking supplements.[276]

"Selenium supplementation of 140 or more µg/day after diagnosis of nonmetastatic prostate cancer may increase risk of prostate cancer mortality. Caution is warranted regarding usage of such supplements among men with prostate cancer," the study warned, effectively proving the previous warning.

A simple blood test will tell you where your selenium levels are, based on your current diet, although interestingly a major review on selenium and prostate cancer found lab tests on fingernail clippings were a more accurate measure of selenium levels than blood tests.[277]

Taking a selenium supplement daily has also been linked to increased risk of oral, head and neck cancers,[278] and several major clinical trials have found a daily selenium supplement boosts your risk of skin cancer by between 40 to 50%.[279] [280]

The New Zealand Nutrition Foundation website helpfully points out that men and women need 60-70 micrograms of selenium a day, and ordinary diet provides it through foods like these:

---

276 "Selenium Supplementation and Prostate Cancer Mortality," Kenfield et al, JNCI *J Natl Cancer Inst* (2015) 107 (1): dju360 doi: 10.1093/jnci/dju360

277 "Selenium and Prostate Cancer: Analysis of Individual Participant Data From Fifteen Prospective Studies," Allen et al, JNCI *J Natl Cancer Inst* (2016) 108 (11): djw153 doi: 10.1093/jnci/djw153

278 Li et al (2012) Vitamin or mineral supplement intake and the risk of head and neck cancer: pooled analysis in the INHANCE consortium. *Int J Cancer* 131: 1686-1689.

279 M. E. Reid, A. J. Duffield-Lillico, E. Slate et al., "The nutritional prevention of cancer: 400Mcg per day selenium treatment," *Nutrition and Cancer,* vol. 60, no. 2, pp. 155-163, 2008.

280 M. Vinceti, G. Dennert, C. M. Crespi et al., "Selenium for preventing cancer," *The Cochrane Database of Systematic Reviews,* vol. 3, Article ID CD005195, 2014.

Foods rich in Selenium	(ug)
1 brazil nut	48
1 poached egg	21
1/2 baked hoki fillet	84
100g tuna (in water)	47
1 grilled fillet steak	21
1 cup natural muesli	13
1 cup cooked pasta	26

How much do we need to eat?

A diet rich in the foods above should meet the selenium needs of most people. You can easily get all the selenium you need from just one Brazil nut, but it is best not to eat more than 2 or 3 per day on a regular basis to avoid selenium toxicity.[281]

Vitamin E

Highly prevalent in vegetable oils, vitamin E is widely used in sunscreens and skin cosmetics, and linked to causing lung and prostate cancer.[282] *Dietary* vitamin E has been linked to a slight protection from cancer, but high use of *supplements* is linked to a 71% increased risk of oral, head and neck cancers [HNC]. Again this raises the question of a balanced holistic diet being better for you than the sum of its parts in a pill.[283]

"Vitamin E supplementation statistically significantly increased the risk of second primary cancers among HNC

---

281   Source: http://www.nutritionfoundation.org.nz/nutrition-facts/minerals/selenium
282 Kristal AR, Darke AK, Morris JS, et al. Baseline selenium status and effects of selenium and vitamin E supplementation on prostate cancer risk. *J Natl Cancer Inst* 2014;106:djt456
283 Li et al, (2012) Vitamin or mineral supplement intake and the risk of head and neck cancer: pooled analysis in the INHANCE consortium. *Int J Cancer* 131: 1686-1689.

patients in a multicenter, double-blind, placebo-controlled, randomized chemoprevention trial," warned a recent review.[284]

What they found was actually surprising. Cancer patients given a daily 400IU dose of vitamin E (alpha tocopherol) for three years during cancer treatment had nearly three times the risk of developing another major cancer during the treatment. Yet if they survived that, their risk of cancer afterwards was reduced by 60%:[285]

"Compared with patients receiving placebo, patients receiving α-tocopherol supplements had a higher rate of second primary cancers during the supplementation period (HR = 2.88, 95% CI = 1.56 to 5.31) but a lower rate after supplementation was discontinued (HR = 0.41, 95% CI = 0.16 to 1.03)."

Moral of the story? If you use vegetable oil in cooking, eat green leafy vegetables, tomatoes, avocadoes, asparagus, broccoli, pumpkin, chicken, dairy, rice or meat, you are probably getting enough vitamin E. Avoid it at all costs in supplements.

Multi Vitamin Tablets

It is often presumed that you can't overdose on multivitamins because their concentrations are low, but beware the wolf in sheep's clothing. One multivitamin tablet a day might be OK and some studies have found them mildly beneficial, but one of those same studies found consumption of *two* multivitamin tablets a day is linked to a 60% increased risk of oral, head and neck cancers.[286]

---

284 ibid
285 Bairati et al, A randomized trial of antioxidant vitamins to prevent second primary cancers in head and neck cancer patients. *J Natl Cancer Inst* 2005; 97: 481-8.
286 Li et al, (2012) Vitamin or mineral supplement intake and the risk of head and neck cancer: pooled analysis in the INHANCE consortium. *Int J Cancer* 131: 1686-1689.

Another study of 13,000 French people given a single multivitamin or a placebo daily for seven years has also raised eyebrows. The daily combination was:

120mg vitamin C
30mg vitamin E
6mg beta-carotene
100mcg selenium
20mg zinc

At the end of the study, women were found to have a 68% higher risk of skin cancer, not a reduced risk as anticipated.[287] Then there's the risk multiplied across each of the ingredients:[288] "Unfortunately, most other studies of vitamin, minerals and other extracted nutrients have shown no benefit, or have actually shown an increased risk of cancer. For example, the CARET study found that beta carotene and retinol [Vitamin A] increased the risk of lung cancer.[289] The Health Professionals Follow-up study (HPFS) which followed the lifestyle habits of 51,529 male professionals for over 15 years found that men who took very high doses of zinc >100mg/day), or took it for long durations were more than twice as likely to develop advanced prostate cancer compared with controls.[290]

---

287 S. Hercberg, K. Ezzedine, C. Guinot et al., "Antioxidant supplementation increases the risk of skin cancers in women but not in men," *Journal of Nutrition*, vol. 137, no. 9, pp. 2098-2105, 2007.
288 Thomas, Robert, et al. "Phytochemicals in cancer prevention and management?." *British Journal of Medical Practitioners* 8.2 (2015). http://bjmp.org/files/2015-8-2/bjmp-2015-8-2-a815.pdf
289 Omenn GS, Goodman GE, Thornquist MD, et al. Risk factors for lung cancer and for intervention effects in CARET, the beta-carotene in retinol efficacy trial. Journal of the National Cancer Institute 1996;88: 1550-1559.
290 Leitzmann MF, Stampfer MJ, Wu K, et al. Zinc supplementation and the risks of prostate

"These data have prompted organisations such as the National Cancer Institute to issue statements stating that long term vitamin and mineral supplements should ideally be given to correct a known deficiency, which is rarely routinely detected unless individuals have self-funded micro-nutrient analysis."

The review notes that while clinical trials on concentrated vitamins and minerals have been disturbing, the news is much better on whole-food extracts, which are concentrations of the entire plant involved, rather than isolated ingredients:

"Studies of concentrated minerals, vitamins and phytoestrogenic [soy] supplements have reported detrimental effects. No study has reported detrimental effects of whole, non-phytoestrogenic food supplements and some have reported significant advantages."

A case in point was the Pomi-T clinical trial, involving whole food extracts of pomegranate, broccoli, green tea and turmeric given to men with prostate cancer. The logic behind it was "to provide a wide spectrum of synergistically acting nutrients, whilst at the same time avoiding over-consumption of one particular phytochemical."[291]

It worked. Compared to placebo, men on the vegetable medley had a 63% reduction in the PSA progression of their cancer.

Another example, and this could be the health tip of the entire book for meat lovers, is that seasoning your meat with rosemary and thyme virtually eliminates cancer-causing chemi-

---

cancer. *Journal of the National Cancer Institute* 2003;95(13): 1004-1007.
291 Thomas, Robert, et al. "Phytochemicals in cancer prevention and management?." *British Journal of Medical Practitioners* 8.2 (2015). http://bjmp.org/files/2015-8-2/bjmp-2015-8-2-a815.pdf

cals known as "HCAs" produced during the cooking process. HCAs are believed responsible for the carcinogenic effects of a meat diet, but it turns out that including plant antioxidants in the roasting dish neutralises the carcinogens:[292]

"Heterocyclic amines (HCAs) in foods have been in the spotlight for many years," food chemistry professor J. Scott Smith said in a news release issued by the Food Safety Consortium and the University of Arkansas agriculture division. "They are carcinogenic and mutagenic compounds that are found at parts per billion levels in cooked fish and meats."

Previous research has shown that grilled beef is a major source of dietary HCAs when cooked at temperatures from 375 degrees F (190.5 degrees C) and above.

"Cooking meats with natural antioxidants decreases or eliminates HCAs on meat," Smith said. Consumers have responded favourably to natural food products in recent years, including natural spices, such as rosemary, which are rich in antioxidants.

Smith's research group began experimenting with marinades containing herbs and spices, notably those related from the mint family such as basil, mint, rosemary, sage, savoury, marjoram, oregano, and thyme. Most of these herbs are rich in three compounds "carnosic acid, carnosol and rosmarinic acid" that are potent antioxidants.

---

292 Smith JS and The Food Safety Consortium. Brush on the marinade, hold off the cancerous compounds. *ScienceDaily* 2007;June 28.

> *"We believe that addition of various substances to the meat before cooking may reduce the carcinogenic HCAs," Smith said. "Marinating steak before grilling is a practical way to reduce HCA contents of even well-done beef for many consumers."*
>
> *Smith's group measured the HCAs in grilled round steaks and found that after marinating them with a commercial product containing rosemary and thyme, the cooked product's level of reduced HCAs "an 87 percent decrease" correlated to the amount of antioxidants present in the marinades.*

Purely as a sidebar, scientists in 2016 discovered rosemary—or specifically rosmarinic acid—acted as a natural sunscreen to actually repair damage caused by sun exposure:

"RA exerted a significant cytoprotective effect by scavenging intracellular ROS [reactive oxygen] induced by UVB. RA also attenuated UVB-induced oxidative macromolecular damage, including protein carbonyl content, DNA strand breaks, and the level of 8-isoprostane. Furthermore, RA increased the expression and activity of superoxide dismutase, catalase, heme oxygenase-1, and their transcription factor Nrf2, which are decreased by UVB radiation. Collectively, these data indicate that RA can provide substantial cytoprotection against the adverse effects of UVB radiation by modulating cellular antioxidant systems, and has potential to be developed as a medical agent for ROS-induced skin diseases."[293]

---

[293] Fernando, Pattage Madushan Dilhara Jayatissa, et al. "Rosmarinic acid attenuates cell damage against UVB radiation-induced oxidative stress via enhancing antioxidant effects in human HaCaT cells." *Biomolecules & therapeutics* 24.1 (2016): 75. doi: 10.4062/

A major review of antioxidant clinical trials published 2015 laments the failure of multi-supplements to protect us from cancer, and particularly the increased risk of tumours in many trials. They have a theory that it is all about balance, not blitzkrieg. Dietary amounts of beta carotene, for example, have been found to protect, whereas high dose concentrated supplements have caused cancers to grow[294]. A research team specifically looking at that wrote:

"The photoprotective effect of beta-carotene reported earlier by others…might depend on interaction with other dietary factors that are either absent, or present in ineffectual concentrations."[295]

It was findings like that which prompted the 2015 review to declare:[296]

"Large RCTs of 4 specific AO [antioxidant] supplements have not shown efficacy. While research is underway on the potential of other AO supplements, and combinations of AO supplements, it is imperative that future studies also target interventions that integrate dietary AOs in the form of whole foods.

"It is well recognized that there is a complex interplay of nutrients present in naturally occurring foods. In consuming

---

biomolther.2015.069

294 C. Liu, X.-D. Wang, R. T. Bronson, D. E. Smith, N. I. Krinsky, and R. M. Russell, "Effects of physiological versus pharmacological β-carotene supplementation on cell proliferation and histopathological changes in the lungs of cigarette smoke exposed ferrets," *Carcinogenesis,* vol. 21, no. 12, pp. 2245-2253, 2000.

295 H. S. Black and J. Gerguis, "Modulation of dietary vitamins E and C fails to ameliorate β-carotene exacerbation of UV carcinogenesis in mice," *Nutrition and Cancer,* vol. 45, no. 1, pp. 36-45, 2003.

296 "Diet and Skin Cancer: The Potential Role of Dietary Antioxidants in Nonmelanoma Skin Cancer Prevention," Rajani Katta and Danielle Nicole Brown, *Journal of Skin Cancer* Volume 2015, Article ID 893149, 10 pages http://dx.doi.org/10.1155/2015/893149

a diet based on whole foods, the finely balanced proportion of nutrients, the large number of potentially protective compounds, and the other plant constituents (such as fibre) may all be necessary.

"Some compounds may potentiate the effects of others, and the role of synergy may make the whole more powerful than the sum of its parts. While there has historically been a focus on the effects of isolated nutrients in human subjects, it is just as vital, if not more so, to continue to study the effects of the entire package of interacting nutrients and substances found in whole foods."

A French review sounded similar warnings:[297]

"In the SU.VI.MAX trial, supplemented women had a significantly increased risk of skin cancer; an increased incidence of prostate cancer was suggested in men with elevated prostate-specific antigen at baseline. These results raise concern that antioxidant supplementation, even at low doses, could have adverse effects on subjects at high risk or with yet undiagnosed cancer. Thus, in a public health approach, it clearly appears more cautious to recommend a lifelong healthy diet including a high consumption of fruits and vegetables, able to provide the antioxidants required, rather than uncontrolled antioxidant supplement use."

Moral of the story? It is the synergy of what we eat that keeps us healthy, not pills. Toxins can often be neutralised by other ingredients in a balanced meal. If you are spending money on

---

297 S. Hercberg, E. Kesse-Guyot, N. Druesne-Pecollo et al., "Incidence of cancers, ischemic cardiovascular diseases and mortality during 5-year follow-up after stopping antioxidant vitamins and minerals supplements: a postintervention follow-up in the SU.VI.MAX Study," *International Journal of Cancer*, vol. 127, no. 8, pp. 1875-1881, 2010. DOI: 10.1002/ijc.25201

an ordinary daily multivitamin, you probably shouldn't or you could cut down your dosage. You will save the cost of this book very quickly, even after buying another copy for a friend, and go on to build up quite a nest-egg moving forward. Not only that, it could save your life given the emerging links between multi-vitamins and cancer.

Instead, look for supplements based on whole food extracts, and look at tweaking your diet. If you think you have a vitamin deficiency or an inability to absorb a vitamin, see your doctor, get it tested.

Astaxanthin

Astaxanthin is another antioxidant that's a rising star in lab tests. Reportedly 100 times better than vitamin E against lipid peroxidation, and 550 times more powerful than vitamin E at soaking up a potent free radical known as 'singlet oxygen', astaxanthin is a marine nutrient that gives shrimp, crayfish, salmon and red snapper their colour. It is also found in flamingos. The good news is that it is also produced by plentiful marine algae.

Unlike some other antioxidants we've examined in this book, astaxanthin has good bioavailability, coupled with strong anti-oxidant, anti-inflammatory and cell-preserving abilities, and "these properties allow astaxanthin to do a lot in the body," says one recent review.[298] "Since it is fat-soluble [it] can be carried by fat molecules [cholesterol] directly to tissues and organs that need it the most, like the brain, retina, and skeletal muscle...

---

298 "Review: Astaxanthin as a Potential Neuroprotective Agent for Neurological Diseases", Wu et al, *Marine Drugs* 2015, 13, 5750-5766; doi:10.3390/md13095750

Astaxanthin is safe to consume with food and contains no reports of side effects."

Like rosemary, and chocolate as we saw in an earlier chapter, astaxanthin also appears to be a potent protection against sun damage to your skin. The aforementioned 'singlet oxygen' is created in the skin by sunlight, so astaxanthin is far more powerful than vitamin E in this regard. In one experiment, esterified astaxanthin in their diets cut the incidence of UV-induced skin cancers in rats by 96%, good reason to include astaxanthin in your own diet.

"UV-DMBA has been known to generate high levels of free radicals and tyrosinase enzyme, leading to characteristic symptoms of skin pigmentation and tumour initiation. Intriguingly, ~7-fold increase in tyrosinase and 10-fold decrease in antioxidant levels were *normalized* by AXDE [astaxanthin diester] and AXME [astaxanthin monoester]."[299]

Still on that theme of repairing sun damage, a series of randomised controlled human trials have confirmed that an oral daily dose of 6mg and topical skin application of 2ml make your skin more youthful, removing wrinkles and age spots.

"Significant improvements as a deep impact were observed in skin wrinkle (crow's feet at week-8), age spot size (cheek at week-8), elasticity (crow's feet at week-8), skin texture (cheek at week-4), moisture content of corneocyte layer (cheek in 10 dry skin subjects at week-8) and corneocyte condition (cheek at week-8)."[300]

---

299 "Effective Inhibition of Skin Cancer, Tyrosinase, and Antioxidative Properties by Astaxanthin and Astaxanthin Esters from the Green Alga Haematococcus pluvialis," Rao et al, dx.doi.org/10.1021/jf304609j | *J. Agric. Food Chem.* 2013, 61, 3842–3851

300 "Cosmetic benefits of astaxanthin on human subjects," Tominaga et al, *Acta Biochimica Polonica* Vol. 59, No 1/2012 43-47

The governing body for cosmetic science product claims in Japan—home to many major cosmetic brands—allows a claim to be made if a significant improvement can be proven in one study parameter. In this case, across two studies, there were improvements in six parameters. Astaxanthin is an anti-aging product, and it works on men as well as women. It is not 'covering up' wrinkles—it is reversing the damage.

According to the scientific journals, 47% of all anticancer drugs used in medicine are sourced from nature, and if you take into account pharmaceutical synthetics of natural compounds, the figure rises to 70%. With most of the big cancers having an up to 20 year lead-time between the first cellular abnormalities in your body and the eventual diagnosis of a tumour, a lot of attention is now being paid to new natural compounds that could slow down or stop that 20 year creep to cancer if we changed our liestyles or diets, or took the 'magic bullet'.

Some cancers are initially triggered by an infection, others by inflammation of tissue caused by irritants and free radicals. In keeping with the theme of this book, it's all about balance because sometimes inflammation is a good thing:[301]

"The innate immune system, in response to harmful stimuli, such as pathogens, dead cells or irritants, starts defence programs to repair damaged tissue. Insufficient inflammation can result in persistent infection by pathogens, while excessive inflammation can cause chronic inflammatory pathologies, including arthritis, diabetes, inflammatory bowel disease, or skin diseases."

---

301 Talero, Elena, et al. "Bioactive compounds isolated from microalgae in chronic inflammation and cancer." *Marine Drugs* 13.10 (2015): 6152-6209.

This is what you are up against, every day. And this is where powerful antioxidants do their thing.

"Astaxanthin has a unique molecular structure which enables it to stay both in and outside the cell membrane. It gives better protection than β-carotene and Vitamin C which can be positioned inside the lipid bilayer. It serves as a safeguard against oxidative damage by various mechanisms, like quenching of singlet oxygen; scavenging of radicals to prevent chain reactions; preservation of membrane structure by inhibiting lipid peroxidation; enhancement of immune system function and regulation of gene expression ."[302]

As previously mentioned, you are not permitted to deliberately infect humans with cancer-causing chemicals to experiment on them (well, not unless you call it 'processed food manufacturing'), but you can with rats.

In a major experiment on astaxanthin's ability to kill colorectal cancer (CRC) in living creatures, a group of rats were studied. Some stayed on a control diet, others were fed astaxanthin. Some were fed a carcinogen known to cause CRC.

Those rats who had been on the astaxanthin supplements before being infected with cancer were able to resist it, and the damage caused by cancer was literally repaired:[303]

"Well-differentiated signs of dysplasia were observed in colonic tissue sections due to DMH induction [infection with carcinogen] that was restored to normalcy in astaxanthin pre-treated rats. The

302 "Astaxanthin: Sources, Extraction, Stability, Biological Activities and Its Commercial Applications–A Review," Ambati et al, *Mar. Drugs* 2014, 12, 128-152; doi:10.3390/md12010128

303 Prabhu, P.N.; Ashokkumar, P.; Sudhandiran, G. Antioxidative and antiproliferative effects of astaxanthin during the initiation stages of 1,2-dimethyl hydrazine-induced experimental colon carcinogenesis. *Fund. Clin. Pharmacol.* 2009, 23, 225-234.

ability of astaxanthin to restore the histological changes induced by DMH indicates the anti-carcinogenic potential of this carotenoid."

Another study looked at how astaxanthin targets cancer cells, and boldly stated: "The results provide compelling evidence that astaxanthin exerts chemopreventive effects ...inducing intrinsic apoptosis. Astaxanthin targets key molecules in oncogenic signalling pathways...and is a promising candidate agent for cancer prevention and therapy."[304]

Clinical trials have shown astaxanthin on its own has no impact on cholesterol levels, although again that may no longer be relevant. It does appear to lower glucose levels slightly.[305]

However, when taken with omega-3 fish oils (that 'whole food' synergy again), the combination delivers a bigger punch than either of its ingredients separately:[306]

"Dietary oils may enhance the absorption of astaxanthin. Astaxanthin with combination of fish oil promoted hypolipidemic/hypocholesterolemic effects in plasma and its increased phagocytic activity of activated neutrophils when compared with astaxanthin and fish oil alone. Astaxanthin was superior to fish oil in particular by improving immune response and lowering the risk of vascular and infectious diseases."

Scientists say animal experiments have proven astaxanthin protects the heart:[307]

---

304 Astaxanthin inhibits NF-κB and Wnt/β-catenin signaling pathways via inactivation of Erk/MAPK and PI3K/Akt to induce intrinsic apoptosis in a hamster model of oral cancer," Kavitha et al, *Biochimica et Biophysica Acta* 1830 (2013) 4433-4444

305 Ursoniu, Sorin, et al. "Lipid profile and glucose changes after supplementation with astaxanthin: a systematic review and meta-analysis of randomized controlled trials." *Arch Med Sci* 11.2 (2015): 253-66. DOI: 10.5114/aoms.2015.50960

306 Ambati et al, *Mar. Drugs* 2014, 12, 128-152; doi:10.3390/md12010128

307 "Review: Astaxanthin: A Potential Therapeutic Agent in Cardiovascular Disease," Robert G. Fassett and Jeff S. Coombes, *Mar. Drugs* 2011, 9, 447-465; doi:10.3390/md9030447

"Experimental studies in several species using an ischaemia-reperfusion myocardial model demonstrated that astaxanthin protects the myocardium when administered both orally or intravenously prior to the induction of the ischaemic event. At this stage we do not know whether astaxanthin is of benefit when administered after a cardiovascular event and no clinical cardiovascular studies in humans have been completed and/or reported. Cardiovascular clinical trials are warranted based on the physicochemical and antioxidant properties, the safety profile and preliminary experimental cardiovascular studies of astaxanthin."

As another major review points out:

"Of several naturally occurring carotenoids, astaxanthin is considered one of the best carotenoids being able to protect cells, lipids and membrane lipoproteins against oxidative damage."[308]

Astaxanthin remains stable at cooking temperatures, and 165gm of salmon will deliver a 3.6mg dose of the nutrient. In one sense it is everything that resveratrol is not. The difference between them is the bioavailability. Both are potent antioxidants, but one hangs around in the system long enough to make a difference. One gives you a quick energy boost and strengthens bones, the other offers sustained protection and appears to be an elixir of youth.

Zeaxanthin And Lutein

Zeaxanthin, another crucial antioxidant, is yellow in colour and takes its name from the botanical name for corn, *Zea mays*. It is also present in high amounts in spirulina. Egg yolks

---

308 "Astaxanthin: Sources, Extraction, Stability, Biological Activities and Its Commercial Applications–A Review," Ambati et al, *Mar. Drugs* 2014, 12, 128-152; doi:10.3390/md12010128

are another good source, in fact laboratory tests have revealed eggs—an animal product—have the highest bioavailability of zeaxanthin in the food chain, whereas it is harder to absorb from plants. One egg a day for five weeks raised serum levels of zeaxanthin in humans by an average 38%, and lutein levels by 26%.[309]

So what do they do? They appear to be critical for eye health. Age-related macular degeneration (AMD) is the leading cause of blindness and there is no cure. But zeaxanthin and lutein have been found in retinal tissue in areas that filter harmful blue light—the kind of light emitted by computer and TV screens, smartphones, tablets, mercury-filled CFLs and LED lights. There is evidence that we are about to face a blue light blindness tsunami in the near future, with teenagers presenting with eye damage previously seen in the elderly. The only thing standing in the way may be zeaxanthin and lutein.

They are believed to soak up free radicals in the eyes, so a diet low in these two nutrients is a step closer to having a guide dog.

A 2014 meta analysis of human clinical trials showed supplementation with lutein and zeaxanthin had "remarkable benefit" in terms of visual acuity, contrast sensitivity and glare recovery time—all key indicators that your eyes are degenerating:[310]

"Lutein and zeaxanthin supplementation is a safe strategy for improving visual performance of AMD patients, which mainly showed in a dose-response relationship."

---

309 E.S.M. Abdel-Aal, H. Akhtar, K. Zaheer, R. Ali, Dietary sources of lutein and zeaxanthin carotenoids and their role in eye health, *Nutrients* 5 (2013) 1169-1185.
310 R. Liu, T. Wang, B. Zhang, L. Qin, C. Wu, Q. Li, L. Ma, Lutein and zeaxanthin supplementation and association with visual function in age-related macular degeneration, *Invest. Ophthalmol. Vis. Sci.* 56 (2014) 252-258.

Manuka Honey

When the superbug revolution finally overpowers medical science, you are going to want a tub of medical grade manuka honey sitting in your kitchen pantry. It has a pedigree:

"Honey," writes the University of Waikato's Peter Molan—a pioneer in honey research—"was used by the ancient Egyptians, Assyrians, Chinese, Greeks and Romans to treat wounds and diseases of the gut. Its use for the treatment of diarrhoea was recommended by the Muslim prophet Mohammed. Aristotle wrote of honey being a salve for wounds and sore eyes and Dioscorides c.50 AD wrote of honey being 'good for all rotten and hollow ulcers'."[311]

Germ theory in modern times is less than 200 years old, but while the ancients may not have known the specifics they instinctively turned to a natural antibiotic to treat infections.

"The use of honey to treat infections has continued into present-day folk-medicine," writes Molan. "In India, lotus honey is traditionally used to treat eye diseases; in Ghana to treat infected leg ulcers; in Nigeria to treat earache; in Mali it is applied on the spots of measles, and in the eyes in measles to prevent scarring of the cornea.

"Honey also has a traditional usage for the treatment of gastric ulcers. Its ancient usage to treat sore throats has continued into the traditional medicine of modern times."

A wide range of honeys from around the world display antibacterial powers, but most do so via hydrogen peroxide. Manuka honey, specifically the New Zealand variety, has an

---

311 http://www.aniwell-uk.com/files/4614/3519/6994/Pdf_6_ANTIBACTERIAL_ ACTIVITY_-libre.pdf

added pathway to killing disease, methylglyoxal, that gives it extra punch.

Methylglyoxal is produced in plants under stress. Because manuka scrub in New Zealand generally grows on land considered too unsuitable to farm, it is believed the manuka generates the stress chemical and bees harvest it as part of the pollen. A New Zealand study compared different honeys from there. The largest concentration of methylglyoxal in a NZ honey was 828mg/kg. In contrast the strongest European honey previously tested had less than 6mg/kg.[312] That's why manuka honey is different.[313]

"Honey is usually derived from the nectar of flowers and produced by bees, most commonly the European honey bee *Apis mellifera,* and is a complex mix of sugars, amino acids, phenolics, and other substances," reports a 2016 review. [314]

"Honey types derived from different flowering plants vary substantially in their ability to kill bacteria, and this has complicated the literature on honey and made it sometimes difficult to reproduce results across different studies."

Manuka honey comes from a scraggly bush native to New Zealand and Australia.

In a twist that may not be a surprise if you have read this book closely in regard to the synergy of whole foods, methylglyoxan can "theoretically be toxic to mammalian cells (Kalapos, 2008). However, there is no evidence of damage to host cells when manuka honey is either consumed orally or used as a wound dress-

---

312 Weigel, K. U.; Opitz, T.; Henle, T. *Eur. Food Res. Technol.* 2004, 218, 147-151.
313 Adams, C. J. et al., *Carbohydr. Res.* (2008), doi:10.1016/j.carres.2007.12.011
314 Carter DA, Blair SE, Cokcetin NN, Bouzo D, Brooks P, Schothauer R and Harry EJ (2016) Therapeutic Manuka Honey: No Longer So Alternative. *Front. Microbiol.* 7:569. doi: 10.3389/fmicb.2016.00569

ing; indeed honey appears to stimulate healing and reduce scarring when applied to wounds. How it exerts this apparently selective toxicity to bacterial cells is not known," noted the 2016 review.

A Welsh study has found manuka honey defeats *Streptococcus pyogenes*, a throat and nasal bacteria that can end up infecting skin wounds in hospitals making them incredibly hard to heal. A 2008 study found nearly 1.5% of people in the developed world have a "non healing wound", being a skin infection that hasn't cleared up within three months. Incredibly, between two and four percent of the health budget is spent trying to clear up these infections every year.[315]

In case you find that hard to fathom, around one in every eight people admitted to a US hospital each day will acquire a hard-to-treat infection in hospital. The average cost to treat is US$54,000 a patient.[316] One in four of these infections will be a wound that won't heal.[317]

Two centuries ago, such wounds were common—and fatal. If your immune system did not overcome the bug, gangrene and amputation, or sepsis and death, were sure to follow.

Then came the discovery of antibiotics—natural bactericides that killed infections. Suddenly, the days of leeches and poultices and 'tut-tutting' in draughty candlelit hallways with a tip 'o the top hat goodnight, were gone. Suddenly, pharmacists were respected, and doctors were no longer 'quacks'. The Golden Age of modern medicine had arrived.

---

315 Gottrup, F. (2008). Trends in surgical wound healing. *Scand J Surg* 97, 220-225, discussion 225-226.
316 Youssef et al, *Dermato-Endocrinology*, Vol 4 Issue 2, Apr-June 2012
317 Werdin et al, (2009). Evidence-based management strategies for treatment of chronic wounds. *Eplasty* 9, e19.

Yet what a difference a few decades make. Today, the shadow of the Bug is back and once again people are actually dying from 'just a scratch'.

Some hard to treat bacteria are not superbugs in the sense that they are resistant to antibiotics. Instead, they have a different weapon in their armour: biofilm. Biofilm is a rapidly multiplying layer of bacteria that forms over a wound site and binds itself to human tissue proteins. By sheer weight of numbers and its chemistry, it becomes very hard for traditional drugs to get rid of.

However, the Welsh trial found medical grade manuka honey killed the Strep infection within eight hours. Not eight days. Eight hours. And so far, despite decades of experiments, no honey-resistant bacteria have ever emerged. Scientists say the honey did not just kill the infection, it also tied its hands behind its back:[318]

"This is the first time that a topical antimicrobial of any type, including manuka honey has been documented to inhibit bacterial binding to a host protein.

"Unlike systemic antibiotics and other topical antimicrobials, the risk of bacterial resistance to manuka honey was low, even when high usage was maintained and to date, no 'honey-resistant' isolates have been found (Blair et al., 2009; Cooper et al., 2010).

"Therefore, manuka honey represents an efficacious and safe alternative to failing systemic and topical treatments that are currently used to treat wounds that are infected with S. pyogenes."

Scientists have actually deliberately tried to create honey-

---

318 "Manuka honey inhibits the development of Streptococcus pyogenes biofilms and causes reduced expression of two fibronectin binding proteins," Maddocks et al, *Microbiology* (2012), 158, 781-790 DOI 10.1099/mic.0.053959-0

resistant superbugs in biosecurity labs, but they have failed. If you have an infection anywhere you can rub, manuka honey can probably kill it:[319]

"Honey has been tested *in vitro* on a diverse range of pathogens," notes the 2016 review, "particularly those that can colonize the skin, wounds and mucosal membranes, where topical honey treatment is possible. To date, in vitro assays have found manuka honey can effectively inhibit all problematic bacterial pathogens tested (summarized in Table1). Of particular interest is that clinical isolates with multiple drug resistance (MDR) phenotypes have no reduction in their sensitivity to honey, indicating a broad spectrum of action that is unlike any known antimicrobial."

The misleadingly-named "Table 1" referred to in the quote actually runs across 4 A4 pages, and lists approximately 60 different bacterial strains including all the known superbugs. If you want to read the full schedule, copy the DOI number listed in the footnote into Google and it will find the document instantly.

An Indian study found 5mls of UMF +19 manuka honey each day, used as a mouth rinse twice daily, slashed the number of tooth decay bacteria in the mouth. Dentists have been leery of recommending honey because of its high sugar content, but the purpose of this study was to see whether those fears were valid. All children in the study also continued to brush their teeth twice daily as well.

Firstly, they found, not all honeys are created equal. It takes

---

319 Carter DA, Blair SE, Cokcetin NN, Bouzo D, Brooks P, Schothauer R and Harry EJ (2016) Therapeutic Manuka Honey: No Longer So Alternative. *Front. Microbiol.* 7:569. doi: 10.3389/fmicb.2016.00569

five times as much non-manuka honey (and therefore more sugar) to kill the bacteria that manuka honey does. Manuka's power-to-weight ratio means it is overall good for the teeth, despite the sugar. The same *Streptococci* bacteria are responsible for gum disease and other oral hygiene issues:[320]

"Children using manuka honey showed statistically significant reductions in salivary *S. mutans* after 10 and 21 days. Conclusion: Manuka honey with UMF 19.5 may be considered as an effective adjunctive oral hygiene measure for reducing colony counts in children."

The study went so far as to suggest children's candy should be manufactured using high UMF honey rather than processed sugar, so their sweets can fight tooth decay while they're being sucked.

The five mls of honey can also be diluted in quarter of a cup of hot water then cooled, to use as a mouthwash.

It's not just antibacterial. Honey is also a fungicide and antiviral. If you have a case of chickenpox or shingles (caused by the varicella zoster virus), recent studies indicate manuka honey may be a viable treatment option.[321]

"Manuka and clover honeys were used at concentrations ranging from 0-6% wt/vol...Both types of honey showed antiviral activity against varicella zoster virus with an approximate $EC_{50} = 4.5\%$ (wt/vol).

"Our results showed that honey has significant in vitro anti-VZV activity. As honey is convenient for skin application, is

320 Rupesh S, Winnier J J, Nayak U A, Rao A P, Reddy N V, Peter J. Evaluation of the effects of manuka honey on salivary levels of mutans streptococci in children: A pilot study. *J Indian Soc Pedod Prev Dent* 2014;32:212-9 DOI: 10.4103/0970-4388.135827
321 Shahzad, A., and Cohrs, R.J. (2012). In vitro antiviral activity of honey against varicella zoster virus (VZV): a translational medicine study for potential remedy for shingles. *Transl. Biomed.* 3:2. DOI: 10.3823/434

readily available and inexpensive, honey may be an excellent remedy to treat zoster rash in developing countries where antiviral drugs are expensive or not easily available."

Honey has been used successfully to treat genital herpes, in fact honey is twice as powerful as acyclovir:[322]

"For genital herpes, the mean duration of attacks and pain, occurrence of crusting, and mean healing time with honey treatment were 53%, 50%, 49% and 59% better, respectively, than with acyclovir... No side effects were observed with repeated applications of honey, whereas 3 patients developed local itching with acyclovir.

"Topical honey application is safe and effective in the management of the signs and symptoms of recurrent lesions from labial and genital herpes."

More proof that honey may be a powerful antiviral came from a 2014 experiment involving influenza in the lab.

Honey was found to inhibit the replication of the influenza virus in a Petri dish. While the chances of honey, influenza and a Petri dish being inside a real patient at any one time are pretty slim, the point is that honey clearly had antiviral strength. Not only that, but it made anti-flu drugs a thousand times more effective when taken with honey.

"Manuka honey efficiently inhibited influenza virus replication, which is related to its virucidal effects. In the presence of 3.13 mg/mL manuka honey, the IC_{50} of zanamivir or oseltamivir was reduced to nearly 1/1000th of their single use. Our results showed that honey, in general, and particularly manuka

---

322 *Med Sci Monit.* 2004 Aug;10(8):MT94-8. Epub 2004 Jul 23. Topical honey application vs. acyclovir for the treatment of recurrent herpes simplex lesions. Al-Waili NS.

honey, has potent inhibitory activity against the influenza virus, demonstrating a potential medicinal value."[323]

The "IC50" is the concentration of a drug necessary to halve the activity of whatever it is targeting. It's a benchmark that scientists use to work out how strong medications need to be. In this case honey massively lowered the necessary dosage of antiviral drugs used with it.

If the world goes to hell in a handcart, stock up on manuka honey.

In the numerous studies done on the topical application of honey to wounds and burns, one thing has become very clear to researchers: it's anti-inflammatory:[324]

"Evidence of reparative activity was seen in 80 per cent of wounds treated with the honey dressing by the 7th day with minimal inflammation. Fifty two per cent of the silver sulfadiazine treated wounds showed reparative activity with inflammatory changes by the 7th day. Reparative activity reached 100 per cent by 21 days with the honey dressing and 84 per cent with SSD. Thus in honey dressed wounds, early subsidence of acute inflammatory changes, better control of infection and quicker wound healing was observed."

Inflammation in tissue is believed to cause cancer and other chronic illnesses. It's one thing to see honey reduce inflammation when applied directly, but what impact does it have when taken on toast and digested?

323 Watanabe, K., Rahmasari, R., Matsunaga, A., Haruyama, T., and Kobayashi, N. (2014). Anti-influenza viral effects of honey in vitro: potent high activity of manuka honey. *Arch. Med. Res.* 45, 359-365. doi:10.1016/j.arcmed.2014.05.006

324 "A prospective randomised clinical and histological study of superficial burn wound healing with honey and silver sulfadiazine", M. Subrahmanyam, *Burns,* Volume 24, Issue 2, March 1998, Pages 157-161

Well, for a start, manuka honey's antibacterial powers are topical, rather than digestive. Honey kills the bugs it can directly touch, but honey does not flow through your veins in its raw form and can't reach bugs in the bloodstream. It's great for sore throats because it kills the bacteria on the way down. Honey has other potencies, however, that may be available internally.

It is good for the heart, and diabetics:[325]

"A report in which two buckwheat honey treatments were administered to 37 healthy human adults at the rate of 1.5 g/kg body weight, with corn syrup as control, has demonstrated increased (p < 0.05) plasma total-phenolic content and plasma anti-oxidant. This study has supported the notion that phenolic anti-oxidants from processed honey are bioavailable and that they increase the anti-oxidant activity of plasma. Therefore, they advocated for the substitution of honey in some foods as traditional sweetener for enhanced anti-oxidant defence system in healthy human adults.

"It has been shown that honey intake ameliorates risk factors of metabolic and cardiovascular diseases in patients and healthy individuals at risk. Unlike refined sugars, diabetic patients can safely and harmlessly eat this natural and sweetest sugar (fructose)- containing product, natural honey.

"Recently, researchers have fed male and female rats with honey or sugar (golden syrup) supplemented diet for 12 weeks from 7 days of age to compare their metabolic response, and see if honey is protective against metabolic syndrome. In male

---

325 Vallianou NG, Gounari P, Skourtis A, Panagos J, Kazazis C (2014) Honey and its Anti-Inflammatory, Anti-Bacterial and Anti-Oxidant Properties. *Gen Med* (Los Angel) 2:132. doi: 10.4172/2327-5146.1000132

rats, golden syrup has significantly increased (p<0.05) blood levels of metabolic substrates (glucose and triglycerides); and caused enhanced (p<0.001) visceral adiposity, hypercholesterolemia, hyperinsulinemia, hepatomegaly and fatty liver. These cardiovascular diseases and metabolic diseases' risk factors were not observed in the honey fed rats in this trial.

"Earlier researches from other laboratories and clinical trials further affirmed the metabolic and cardiovascular health significance of eating honey by recording some health profiles. These were reduction in the plasma levels of risk factors which include total cholesterol, LDL-cholesterol, triglycerides, glucose in normal and diabetic patients, C-reactive protein, while the health indices elevated in the blood were HDL cholesterol.

"Besides that, other researchers recorded higher plasma antioxidants levels in rats nurtured with natural honey relative to fructose-fed rats, and consequently low susceptibility of these subjects to cardiovascular diseases. Another study has demonstrated that the combination of glibenclamide or metformin with honey improves glycemic control, and provides additional metabolic benefits, not achieved with either glibenclamide or metformin alone in streptozocin-induced diabetic rats."

A clinical trial in Dubai found honey ingested as part of the diet every day lowered inflammatory prostaglandin levels by up to 63% over the 15 day study.[326]

Honey has been found to attack a wide range of cancer tumours in lab tests, and scientists say there's good reason to

---

326 Natural honey lowers plasma prostaglandin concentrations in normal individuals," Al-Waili, N.S, Boni, N.S, *Journal of Medicinal Food* Volume 6, Issue 2, June 2003, Pages 129-133

believe that a honey diet has strong anticancer action in the body as well.

"Though the full mechanism is yet to be fully understood, studies have shown that honey has anticancer effect through its interference with multiple cell-signalling pathways, such as inducing apoptosis, antiproliferative, anti-inflammatory, and antimutagenic pathways. Honey modulates the body immune system. There are still many unanswered questions; why sugar is carcinogenic, while honey which is basically sugar has anti-carcinogenic properties."[327]

It's that same fundamental question again: what's the synergy that makes this work? Is the brutal truth that food processing by humans cannot come close to natural foods, that our science and chemistry—for all of its high-tech glamour—is but a blunt instrument in comparison to the work of a bee, a cocoa bean, a salmon fillet or a humble mutton chop? Is it true that when so-called "active ingredients" are extracted, that it may simply be guesswork?

Perhaps the bigger question you should be asking is, just how much science and chemistry is going on with our food, and who is behind it?

---

327 Sarfraz Ahmed and Nor Hayati Othman, "Honey as a Potential Natural Anticancer Agent: A Review of Its Mechanisms," *Evidence-Based Complementary and Alternative Medicine,* vol. 2013, Article ID 829070, 7 pages, 2013. doi:10.1155/2013/829070

9

EPILOGUE : Big Pharma's War On Food

Y OU MAY BE wondering just where Big Pharma sits in all this. As alluded to at times in this book, global multinationals are tightening control of food production worldwide, and they now have defacto control of global food regulations.

In late 2013 I revealed just how incestuous the industry is, in my book *Totalitaria*:

The money, the payoff, comes from the implementation of such a system globally because it means the multinationals can carve up the third world markets where most of the growth will come from this century. The real money in controlling the world won't be made in America or New Zealand or the UK—it will be made in Africa, Asia, South America and the Middle East. But those markets can't be fully exploited until a world governance structure is put in place that protects the exploiters from the whims of sovereign countries. Once a country ratifies Codex—like any UN treaty—it is in for life, and subject to crushing trade sanctions if it doesn't obey the rules.

This, of course, plays right into the hands of global multinationals like Dow Agrosciences and Monsanto. Both of these companies are perhaps best known for producing toxic chemicals—herbicides and pesticides.

Monsanto's board of directors includes the head of McDonalds USA, and a top executive with Procter & Gamble.

Despite using the phrase "Sustainable Agriculture" on its website, the company has an exceedingly bad reputation. It manufactured nearly 100% of the toxic PCBs now polluting the USA. Its manufacturing operations in the UK created a toxic waste dump as well. It plays a huge role however in guiding global food, agriculture and chemical rules.

Although Monsanto's corporate website only contains a glancing reference to Codex in two documents, the Codex website contains 379 documents featuring Monsanto. The multinational works through a range of front organisations, like the International Life Sciences Institute, or the Alliance to Feed The Future. These are all "soft faces" for Monsanto PR executives to manipulate the system.

The Alliance, for example, is controlled by an outfit called the International Food Information Council. When you go to the IFIC website, if you know where to dig (it is not easy), you will eventually find it is funded by a group of global multinationals including:[328]

---

328 http://www.foodinsight.org/linkclick.aspx?fileticket=09a8FrY%2bp7M%3d&tabid=91

- Monsanto
- DuPont
- Abbott Nutrition
- Bayer Crop Science
- Dow AgroSciences
- Coca Cola
- Dr Pepper
- General Mills
- Hershey
- Heinz
- Kelloggs
- Kraft
- Mars
- McDonalds
- Nestle
- Pepsi
- Red Bull
- Unilever

The International Food Information Council sees its role as "educating" the public and the media about nutrition and food safety. "We also serve as a news media resource. We provide science-based information to the media and refer journalists to our 350 independent, credentialed experts on a variety of nutrition and food safety topics."[329]

It's a very slick PR campaign, complete with soundbites delivered on the issues of the day to media everywhere.

Its "partners" include a veritable who's who of global food

---

329 http://www.foodinsight.org/about-ific-and-food-safety.aspx

and health organisations. The outlets endorse the IFIC, in fact the American Academy of Physicians Assistants even endorsed a puff piece brochure advising consumers that the artificial sweetener aspartame is perfectly safe:

"Aspartame has been studied extensively and has been found to be safe by experts and researchers. Government agencies worldwide, including the U.S. Food and Drug Administration (FDA), have also reviewed the science and found aspartame to be safe for human consumption."[330]

Aspartame was once one of Monsanto's mainstay products, you may know it better by its trade names NutraSweet and Equal, among others. It is surprising that the statement above about it being "studied extensively" made it through peer review. In 2012 the *American Journal of Clinical Nutrition* published a study linking aspartame use in humans to a higher risk of cancer, and it was critical at how "sparse" previous human studies had been and how poorly designed those studies were, with "only short term follow-up". In simple terms, if you hadn't developed cancer within a short time of drinking diet soda, that proved it was "safe" for the purposes of the food industry.

This new study followed diet soda drinkers for up to 20 years and found the risk of cancer more than doubled for some tumours.[331] Another study of 59,000 Danish pregnant women has found consumption of diet soft drinks strongly increased the risk of having an early premature baby.[332]

330 http://www.foodinsight.org/Content/3848/FINAL_Aspartame%20Brochure_Web%20 Version_11-2011.pdf
331 "Soft drinks, aspartame, and the risk of cancer and cardiovascular disease", Am J Clin Nutr December 2012 vol. 96 no. 6 1249-1251
332 "Intake of artificially sweetened soft drinks and risk of preterm delivery: a prospective cohort study in 59,334 Danish pregnant women", Halldorsson et al, 2010, doi: 10.3945/ajcn.2009.28968 Am J Clin Nutr September 2010 vol. 92 no. 3 626-633

It turns out that virtually all the studies that have found aspartame to be safe were funded by or linked to the interests of aspartame manufacturers—exactly the same shonky science we saw with Big Pharmaceuticals. As Professor Ralph G. Walton, M.D., Professor of Clinical Psychiatry, at the USA's Northeastern Ohio Universities College of Medicine, warned back in 2003: "The diet food industry and the F.D.A. are fond of saying that aspartame is 'the most studied product in history' with an outstanding safety record. In fact however virtually all of the studies in the medical literature attesting to its safety were funded by the industry[333], whereas independently funded studies, now numbering close to 100, identify one or more problems."[334]

Sometimes it isn't additives but residues. For two decades, Monsanto, the chemical giant that manufactures Roundup (glyphosate) has been developing genetically modified food crops, and getting them authorised for use in the food chain. The point of these crops was not modification to make them more nutritious, but to make them more resistant to herbicides—specifically Monsanto's own herbicide Roundup—or in some cases the crops were engineered to produce their own pesticide. For farmers, that means they can dump greater quantities of the weed-killer Roundup on the crops secure in the knowledge it will get rid of the weeds but not kill the crop.

Monsanto wins two ways: firstly, it sells vastly more Roundup. Secondly, it owns the rights to the genetically-modified crop seeds, so that farmers are forced to buy seed from Monsanto each year.

Of more concern, for decades Monsanto has claimed Roundup is safe and wheeled out scientific studies supposedly proving

333 http://www.dorway.com/peerrev.html
334 http://www.thebriefingroom.com/archives/2007/11/aspartame_sweet.html

that. Given the recent revelations about scientific fraud by big pharmaceutical companies, that may be reason for caution. Fears rise considerably when some newer studies are added to the mix. A 2012 study on rats fed Roundup-resistant GM corn found death rates doubled or tripled, thanks to cancer and kidney damage.

"A Roundup-tolerant maize and Roundup provoked chronic hormone and sex dependent pathologies. Female mortality was 2–3 times increased mostly due to large mammary tumors and disabled pituitary. Males had liver congestions, necrosis, severe kidney nephropathies and large palpable tumors. This may be due to an endocrine disruption linked to Roundup and a new metabolism due to the transgene. GMOs and formulated pesticides must be evaluated by long term studies to measure toxic effects."[335]

That study was quickly attacked by official Food Safety agencies in Europe, Australia and New Zealand[336], who claimed the cancers and other rat defects could be explained by natural variation. Given that glyphosate is now the world's most widely-used herbicide, and manufactured by a range of massive multinationals, there is a huge amount riding on this research, and the industry is certainly not standing by to see its golden goose killed off.

The Food Safety agencies are creatures of the United Nations Codex, and Codex and its national agencies—as we have established—have Monsanto and the other massive multinationals as key technical advisors.

Case in point, one of Monsanto's top lawyers, Michael Taylor, was appointed at senior advisor to the Food and Drug Adminis-

---

335 "Long term toxicity of a Roundup herbicide and a Roundup-tolerant genetically modified maize", Seralini et al, Food and Chemical Toxicology, Volume 50, Issue 11, November 2012, Pages 4221–4231
336 http://www.foodstandards.govt.nz/consumer/gmfood/seralini/pages/default.aspx

tration in the US, making him, as the *Huffington Post* reported, "now America's food safety czar. What have we done?"[337]

The *Huff* linked to leaked documents disclosing how Monsanto and the regulators had covered up suspected toxicities in the GM food ranges.[338]

Monsanto and the pharmaceutical giants are owned, for the most part, by exactly the same massive Wall Street investment funds and merchant banks. It is as if western economic power is concentrated in Big Pharma and Big Chemical, and companies like Monsanto, Glaxo or Johnson & Johnson are little more than brand-differentiated sock puppets of the same shareholders.[339]

In plain English: food sprayed with Roundup (which is most commercially produced plant food) appears to be poisonous. The cynical amongst you have probably already realised that if the same shareholders who own the companies poisoning your food also own the companies making expensive medicines, then they are managing to clip the ticket at both ends of the deal.

"Contrary to the current widely-held misconception that glyphosate is relatively harmless to humans, the available evidence shows that glyphosate may rather be the most important factor in the development of multiple chronic diseases and conditions that have become prevalent in Westernized societies," the MIT study notes.

To get an idea of just how big this timebomb could be, consider these US Department of Agriculture figures. In 2000, just

---

337 "You're Appointing Who? Please Obama, Say It's Not So!" by Jeffrey Smith, Huffington Post, 23 July 2009, http://www.huffingtonpost.com/jeffrey-smith/youre-appointing-who-plea_b_243810.html
338 http://biointegrity.org/index.htm
339 Compare shareholdings for Monsanto, Johnson & Johnson and Glaxo here: http://finance.yahoo.com/q/mh?s=MON+Major+Holders and here: http://finance.yahoo.com/q/mh?s=JNJ+Major+Holders and here: http://finance.yahoo.com/q/mh?s=GSK+Major+Holders

7% of the national maize crop was genetically-modified to be Roundup-resistant. By 2012, 73% of corn was Roundup-ready.[340] Another study found farmers were now able to apply between 200 and 500% more Roundup on their crops than they had previously done—five times more of the chemical.

No wonder Monsanto and the other Roundup makers like Dow and Syngenta are smiling.

Some of you right now might be asking, hang on, if the Food Police are being given power to raid your kitchen and squeeze your muffins, surely they have the power to enforce the safety of genetically-modified food? The short answer is no, they don't.[341]

As it currently stands under the UN food Codex that the multinationals are operating under, responsibility for testing the safety of GM food ingredients is left in the hands of the multinationals and their own research labs. There is to be no independent oversight by the Food Police.

"The stance taken by Monsanto, Dow and the other peddlers of both chemicals and genetically engineered seeds is that GMO food is 'identical to non-GMO products'. They claim that genetic engineering is no different than plant hybridization, which has been practiced for centuries. It is the reason they gave, and the EPA accepted, for not having to submit GMO food to rigorous testing to obtain EPA approval. It's up to the companies

---

340 http://www.ers.usda.gov/datafiles/Adoption_of_Genetically_Engineered_Crops_in_the_US/alltables.xls

341 In fact, the US Government snuck in a provision in March 2013 under the cover of a budget bill, that made Monsanto and other big chemical companies legally immune in the event their genetic modification injures the public. It's been dubbed the "Monsanto Protection Act", and specifically is Clause 735 of the bill HR 933 passed on 22 March 2013. As Salon magazine wrote: "The provision protects genetically modified seeds from litigation in the face of health risks…President Barack Obama signed the spending bill, including the provision, into law on Tuesday." For a link to the actual legislation, and the background, see Salon: http://www.salon.com/2013/03/27/how_the_monsanto_protection_act_snuck_into_law/

that manufacture GMOs to research and determine the safety of their products," says GMO expert and commentator Dr Nancy Swanson.[342] She's not a medical doctor, but a retired university physics professor and US Navy scientist.[343]

The idea that genetic modification is the same as cross-breeding and 'hybridization' is something she finds laughable:

"Not only are the bacteria genes [inserted into plants] themselves potentially toxic, but the plants can be sprayed directly with herbicides, the herbicide-resistant plants absorb the poisons and we eat them. It's difficult to understand how this can be considered 'essentially' the same as plant hybridization."

And all of this, without any genuine independent testing of the organisms.

In fact, the Monsanto/Bayer/Dow/DuPont sponsored International Food Information Council boasts about its ability to control its own safety testing under what is known as GRAS, or Generally Regarded As Safe regime.

In a powerpoint presentation, delegates are told that using the GRAS regime to get food additives approved in the US is much faster and simpler than going through the formal petition process with the Food and Drug Administration.

Under a question, "Who makes Safety Determination?", delegates are told:

"Submitter of Notification; Uses Experts; FDA Issues No Objection Letter."[344]

The process takes "days" or "months", compared to "years"

---

342 http://www.examiner.com/article/washington-state-residents-likely-to-vote-on-gmo-food-labels-1
343 http://www.examiner.com/gmo-in-seattle/nancy-swanson
344 http://www.foodadditives.org/pdf/Safety%20and%20Suitability%20of%20Food%20Additives.pdf

under the formal petition process. Of course, if you control the experts, the whole process is plain sailing.

And that's exactly what an independent review has just found. In the *Journal of the American Medical Association* "Internal Medicine" issue in August 2013, researchers found the Food and Drug Administration doesn't even know what many of the food additive chemicals actually are! The GRAS regime dates back to 1958, and it has been used to approve around 43% of the 10,000 chemicals known to have been OK'd for use in food.

What's worse, of those 10,000 chemicals, a thousand of them have never been disclosed to the FDA at all. The FDA is completely in the dark about precisely what those chemicals might be.

The JAMA team analysed 451 GRAS applications made between 1997 and 2012 and published on the FDA's website. What they found shows you just how total the control of the chemical companies is over official food safety—not one of the 451 Generally Regarded As Safe approvals was made by an independent expert. Not one:

"About 22 percent were made by an employee of the food additive manufacturer and about 13 percent by employees of consulting firms hired by manufacturers," reported Reuters.[345]

"Another 64 percent were submitted by food safety expert panels whose members were picked by either manufacturers or consulting firms to evaluate the additive. None of the panels, which included an average of four people, were selected by third parties, the study found.

"Neltner's study also found that 10 experts served on 27 or

---

345 "Industry has "undue influence" over U.S. food additives: study", Reuters, 7 August 2013 http://www.reuters.com/article/2013/08/07/us-food-additives-bias-idUSBRE9760Z820130807

more panels. One of them was a member of 128 panels, about 44 percent of the total."

Another study in the journal *Reproductive Toxicology* surveyed the FDA food additive database and found that there was insufficient toxicology data on 80% of the additives to illustrate what the safe human consumption limits of the chemicals actually are.[346]

In fact, of the 10,000 or so known food chemicals, no controlled safety tests have been done on a large majority, says the new report:

"Almost two-thirds of chemical additives appear to have been declared safe for use in food without the benefit of being fed to an animal in a controlled toxicology study."

What are the implications for the health of you and your family? In short, the chemicals added to processed foods may well be toxic to adults and children, because no real safety data has ever been provided: "given the substantial lack of toxicology data for chemical additives, extrapolation of the limited information to so many chemicals is disconcerting and may be insufficient to ensure safety. Therefore, it may represent a public health problem.

"With almost two-thirds of chemical additives lacking feeding toxicology and 78.4% of additives directly added to food lacking data to estimate a safe level of exposure and 93% lacking reproductive or development toxicity testing, it is problematic to assert that we know with reasonable certainty that all chemical additives are safe.

---

346 "Data gaps in toxicity testing of chemicals allowed in food in the United States", Thomas G. Neltner et al, Reproductive Toxicology, Volume 42, December 2013, Pages 85–94 http://www.sciencedirect.com/science/article/pii/S0890623813003298

"Although FDA is aware of the problem, it lacks the authority and resources to fill the information gaps. Furthermore, once a chemical is approved, manufacturers have no incentive to add additional toxicology information because FDA neither has a reassessment program in place nor has authority to require additional testing."

In response, the Grocery Manufacturers Association in America defended the GRAS system, telling the media it was a "thorough and comprehensive process". Believe that, and you will believe pigs can fly. Given Monsanto's involvement in genetic engineering of pigs, however, that does remain a possibility.

You can read a list of the Food Additive numbers for some of the additives on Wikipedia if you are curious.

These global food industry bodies representing the chemical companies and processed food manufacturers all insist they are "compliant" with the UN's Codex Alimentarius. The shocking thing is, they're not lying, they are compliant with UN edicts because to a large extent they control Codex. They are drafting food laws across the world[347] that heavily favour globalised food processors, but which will heavily punish any homeowners, farmers or small businesses trying to compete by offering more natural food.

It is no coincidence that New Zealand's Codex-compliant Food Bill specifically excluded genetically modified food from

---

347 Among them, the global corporations are united in opposing food product labelling laws. Calfifornia's Prop. 37 law seeking mandatory disclosure of genetically modified content on food labels was opposed by Monsanto, DuPont, Hersheys, Mars, Kraft, PepsiCo and Syngenta, to name a few, who donated tens of millions of dollars to fund advertising campaigns against GM labelling. Their campaign succeeded, voters opted not to support labelling. Similar political/corporate opposition to labelling is found in New Zealand and other Codex-dominated countries. http://www.huffingtonpost.com/2012/11/02/prop-37-donors-revealed-f_n_2065789.html

the items the Food Police have jurisdiction over.[348] It is also no coincidence that these multinational companies make some of the biggest profits on the planet.

To add insult to injury, five years after making a $5 Million donation to the World Food Prize Foundation, Monsanto this year won the event through one of its top GMO scientists, leaving critics speechless:

"Winning this prize will encourage the wider use of genetically engineered crops and be a huge obstacle to those fighting to investigate the long-term effects of its frankenseeds—which is exactly what Monsanto wants," said activist Oliver Moldenhauer. "In 2008, Monsanto made a $5 million pledge to the World Food Prize Foundation, part of its plan to buy the credibility it can't legitimately earn. By handing its benefactor this award, the Foundation risks undermining the credibility of the most respected prize in agriculture."[349]

One of the scientists who shared the prize worked for Syngenta, whose pesticides have been accused in Europe of contributing to the demise of bee colonies.

Do you still trust the United Nations and your national food regulatory agency, or are you beginning to suspect you are being conned?

The way Codex treats natural health supplements like vitamins and minerals stands in sharp contrast to the slack stand-

---

348 After public pressure, the Government agreed in 2013 to include a clause in the Bill permitting the New Zealand government to make its own laws on GM food. This was not included in the original international treaty guiding the process and has to be managed under the "exceptional circumstances" clause of the international treaty. Even so, Food Minister Nikki Kaye says "The Food Bill supports the existing robust scientific pre-approval process required prior to GM foods being allowed for sale". As you have seen, the process is far from "robust". http://www.scoop.co.nz/stories/PA1306/S00184/food-bill-changes-better-balance-legislation.htm
349 http://blogs.vancouversun.com/2013/10/15/consumer-group-outraged-at-monsanto-winning-nobel-prize-of-agriculture/

ards on other food chemicals. While Monsanto, Dow, DuPont and others can sneak chemicals into food with no controlled safety tests whatsoever, they influenced Codex to require full scientific testing of vitamin and mineral supplements, as the Codex guidelines make clear:

"Vitamin and mineral food supplements should contain vitamins/provitamins and minerals whose nutritional value for human beings has been proven by scientific data and whose status as vitamins and minerals is recognised by FAO [UN Food and Agriculture Organisation] and WHO [UN World Health Organisation]."[350]

At the same time, the big players, backed by the US and Food Standards Australia New Zealand (FSANZ), tried to encourage Codex not to cut the food additive aluminium from the approved list. You didn't know you were eating the toxic metal that's been linked to Alzheimers and other nasties? Don't worry, few people do know. One who does is US attorney Scott Tips, the general counsel for the National Health Federation in the US. The NHF is the only accredited consumer watchdog group permitted to attend Codex meetings, and Tips says the battle over aluminium is typical of the struggle.[351]

"Aluminum is a known neurotoxin, easily crossing the blood-brain barrier, and it interferes with ATP enzymes, which carry out the important function of energy transfer among brain cells. Aluminum worsens the effects of other toxins, such as pesticides, herbicides, mercury, cadmium, fluoride, lead, and glutamate. It also detaches highly oxidizing iron in the

---

350 "Guidelines for vitamin and mineral food supplements CAC/GL 55—2005" Codex Alimentarius Commission
351 http://www.newswithviews.com/Tips/scott118.htm

bloodstream from its protective carrier transferrin. This greatly increases the toxicity of iron and is at least one of the mechanisms by which aluminum is toxic to the brain. Warnings about the toxic effects of aluminum could, and do, fill volumes.

"Aluminum ammonium sulfate, aluminum silicate, calcium aluminum silicate, sodium aluminum phosphates, and sodium aluminosilicate are the food additives that Codex was reviewing this session. They can be found in practically as many foods as you can imagine: vegetables, soybean paste, crackers, pastas and noodles, bagels, English muffins, pita bread, bread and baking mixes, chewing gum, milk and cream powder, processed cheeses, flours, batters for fish and poultry, dairy-based drinks such as eggnog, beverage whiteners, dried-whey products, salt, seasonings and condiments, soup and broth mixes, and sauces. And do not think that you can always look at labels and see them disclosed there because often the aluminum compound is hidden within a particular product identity."

The Aluminum Association of American discloses on its website that it was not happy when NHF managed to get the tolerable weekly limit of aluminium intake for humans lowered from 7mg a week to 1mg, per kilogram of body weight.

"In June of 2006, the Codex scientific group, JECFA, lowered the PTWI for aluminum from all sources from 7mg/kgbw to 1mg/kgbw. The aluminum industry has actively engaged the JECFA to re-assess the PTWI, based on new research completed by the industry to comply with emerging global regulations.

"A coalition of associations representing both aluminum producers and food additives manufacturers has completed research addressing data gaps that led to the downward revision of the PTWI and will present that research to the Codex group," said the Aluminum Association to its members in 2011. Their campaign was successful. The tolerable limit of aluminium was doubled to 2mg per kilo of body weight per week, with the approval of the World Health Organisation.[352]

The European Food Safety Authority did its own research in 2008 and revealed children are at highest risk of exposure to aluminium, because of their small body weight but big appetites, and because the metal is present in most processed foods and infant milk formula, where levels reached 0.9 mg/kg of body weight per week for dairy powder, and 1.1mg/kg for soy formula.[353]

Some big brand infant formulas, it noted, contained four times that amount:

"The Panel noted that in some individual brands of formulae (both milk-based and soya-based) the aluminium concentration was around 4 times higher that the mean concentrations estimated above, leading to a 4 times higher potential exposure in brand-loyal infants."

In keeping with the "breast is best" message, aluminium levels were a staggering 63 times lower in breast milk:

"Potential exposure in breast-fed infants was estimated to be less than 0.07 mg/kg bw/week."

The European Food Safety Authority reports that "Aluminium can enter the brain and reach the placenta and fetus," and that it remains in the body for "a very long time in various organs and tissues".

---

352 "WHO Committee Ups Recommended Intake Limit for Aluminum in Diet", Aluminum Association, http://www.aluminum.org/AM/Template.cfm?Section=Weekly_Briefing&Template=/CM/HTMLDisplay.cfm&ContentID=31824
353 "Safety of aluminium from dietary intake: Scientific Opinion of the Panel on Food Additives, Flavourings, Processing Aids and Food Contact Materials (AFC)European Food Safety Authority, 2007 The EFSA Journal (2008) 754, 1-34, http://www.efsa.europa.eu/en/efsajournal/doc/754.pdf

What's interesting is that the EFSA noted that there were next to no studies on the safety of aluminium in human diet, so it opted for an upper limit of 1mg/kgbw per week. It reached that decision in a 122 page report analysing the science. Despite that, the World Health Organisation after lobbying from the aluminium and food additives industry doubled the permissible levels.

It's worth taking a look at what quantities of this toxic metal the United Nations approved for public consumption. Up until 2006, based on the previous 7mg limit, an average 85kg male was absorbing 31 grams of aluminium into his body each year through food, deodorant and a range of other avenues and products. That's around 1.9kg of aluminium you've ingested by the age of 70. And they wonder why dementia sets in.

Under the new limit, someone born today will absorb more than half a kilogram of this metal over their life time.

But here's something else you didn't know: those figures are the "recommended" intake levels. Depending on how much processed food you eat, how much tinfoil you use in your food preparation and the like, your actual exposure each week, according to the EFSA can actually be this high:

"The results ranged from 18.6 to 156.2 mg/kg bw/week at the mean and from 35.3 to 286.8 mg/kg bw/week at the 95th percentile."[354]

As the EFSA forlornly noted, the actual intakes of dietary aluminium "exceed" by an order of magnitude the tolerable limits.

Putting that in plain English, a person at the upper range could absorb *1.27kg of aluminium a year*, or 89kg over a lifetime. That's equivalent to casting a statue of you in aluminium, or auditioning

---

354 "Dietary exposure to aluminium-containing food additives", Question number: EFSA-Q-2013-00312 Issued: 13 March 2013, http://www.efsa.europa.eu/en/supporting/pub/411e.htm

as the Tin Man in the Wizard of Oz. If all that aluminium from just one year was concentrated in one lump in your body you would set off the metal detectors at airports. If it was magnetic, you would be a serious navigational hazard on a plane.

The studies keep mounting up, with one recent animal testing experiment concluding that exposure to aluminium, "particularly during pregnancy and lactation period, can affect the in utero developing fetus and postnatal…raising the concerns that during a critical perinatal period of brain development, Al exposure has potential and long lasting neurotoxic hazards."[355]

Another new study on human brains reinforces the disturbing message:

"Once biologically available aluminum bypasses gastrointestinal and blood–brain barriers, this environmentally-abundant neurotoxin has an exceedingly high affinity for the large pyramidal neurons of the human brain hippocampus. This same anatomical region of the brain is also targeted by the earliest evidence of Alzheimer's disease (AD) neuropathology."[356]

The study reports that "human brain endothelial cells were found to have an extremely high affinity for aluminium", meaning that the food you are feeding yourself or your children, approved by the United Nations Codex and enforced by your local food laws, may be giving you a very nasty death sentence in the form of eventual dementia.

Good to know the chemical companies have been adding

---

355 "Neurobehavioral toxic effects of perinatal oral exposure to aluminum on the developmental motor reflexes, learning, memory and brain neurotransmitters of mice offspring," Gasem M. Abu-Taweela et al, Pharmacology Biochemistry and Behavior, Volume 101, Issue 1, March 2012, Pages 49–56
356 "Selective accumulation of aluminum in cerebral arteries in Alzheimer's disease (AD)" Bhattacharjeea et al, Journal of Inorganic Biochemistry, Volume 126, September 2013, Pages 35–37, http://www.sciencedirect.com/science/article/pii/S0162013413001207

it to our food. Not so good to know that FSANZ downunder and FDA in the USA have been complicit in this. It probably won't come as a surprise to learn that "to this date, aluminum has never been tested for safety by the FDA," says Tips.

So, what's the moral of this entire story?

Some very big food multinationals have made their fortunes for decades pitching their products as 'healthy', when in fact scientific trials are linking those foods to illness and death. Those same food companies in many cases have the same shareholders as the big pharmaceutical giants who profit from the medical treatment you require.

You—Joe and Jane Public—put your trust in government authorities to regulate food safety and advise you on a healthy diet, yet their advice increasingly seems to be at odds with actual scientific test results.

The studies you have read in this book are all from peer-reviewed medical journals. The scientists who carried them out have dared to say, "the Emperor has no clothes".

If you remember nothing else, remember the hamsters. The ones on the diet your doctor recommends died the youngest. The ones eating chocolate and lard lived the longest. Don't be the sad hamster.

If you enjoyed *Show Me The Money, Honey*, leave a review on Amazon.com and Goodreads to help spread the word. Donate a copy to your doctor or a friend or family member. Pay it forward. Change someone's life.

For a fully text-searchable version of this book, download a copy from Amazon, Kobo or your preferred ebook store.